Orthopedic Review

for Undergraduate Students

Orthopedic Review

for Undergraduate Students

Kavin Khatri MS, DNB, FACS

Assistant Professor
Department of Orthopedics
GGS Medical College
Faridkot, Punjab

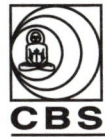

CBS

CBS Publishers & Distributors Pvt Ltd

New Delhi • Bengaluru • Chennai • Kochi • Kolkata • Mumbai
Bhopal • Bhubaneswar • Hyderabad • Jharkhand • Nagpur • Patna • Pune
• Uttarakhand • Dhaka (Bangladesh)

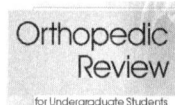

ISBN: 978-93-88527-70-5

First Edition: 2019

Published by Satish Kumar Jain and produced by Varun Jain for
CBS Publishers & Distributors Pvt Ltd
4819/XI Prahlad Street, 24 Ansari Road, Daryaganj, New Delhi 110 002, India.

Ph: 23289259, 23266861, 23266867   Fax: 011-23243014

Website: www.cbspd.com   e-mail: delhi@cbspd.com; cbspubs@airtelmail.in.

Corporate Office: 204 FIE, Industrial Area, Patparganj, Delhi 110 092

Ph: 4934 4934   Fax: 4934 4935

          e-mail: publishing@cbspd.com; publicity@cbspd.com

Branches

- **Bengaluru:** Seema House 2975, 17th Cross, K.R. Road,
  Banasankari 2nd Stage, Bengaluru 560 070, Karnataka
  Ph: +91-80-26771678/79   Fax: +91-80-26771680   e-mail: bangalore@cbspd.com
- **Chennai:** 7, Subbaraya Street, Shenoy Nagar, Chennai 600 030, Tamil Nadu
  Ph: +91-44-26680620, 26681266   Fax: +91-44-42032115   e-mail: chennai@cbspd.com
- **Kochi:** 42/1325, 1326, Power House Road, Opposite KSEB Power House,
  Ernakulam 682 018, Kochi, Kerala
  Ph: +91-484-4059061-65   Fax: +91-484-4059065   e-mail: kochi@cbspd.com
- **Kolkata:** 6/B, Ground Floor, Rameswar Shaw Road, Kolkata-700 014, West Bengal
  Ph: +91-33-22891126, 22891127, 22891128   e-mail: kolkata@cbspd.com
- **Mumbai:** 83-C, Dr E Moses Road, Worli, Mumbai-400018, Maharashtra
  Ph: +91-22-24902340/41   Fax: +91-22-24902342   e-mail: mumbai@cbspd.com

Representatives

• **Bhopal**	0-8319310552	• **Bhubaneswar**	0-9911037372
• **Hyderabad**	0-9885175004	• **Jharkhand**	0-9811541605
• **Nagpur**	0-9021734563	• **Patna**	0-9334159340
• **Pune**	0-9623451994	• **Uttarakhand**	0-9716462459
• **Dhaka (Bangladesh)**	01912-0034853		

Printed at Mudrak, Noida, UP, India

Contributors

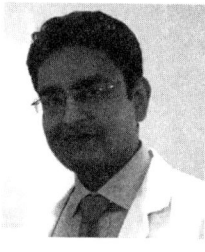

Deepak Bansal MS (Orthopedics)
Consultant, Department of orthopedics
AIMC Bassi Hospital, Tagore Nagar
Ludhiana, Punjab

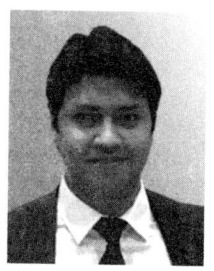

Darsh Goyal MS (Orthopedics)
Consultant, Department of orthopedics
Bhagat Chandra Hospital, Mahavir Enclave
Palam Colony, New Delhi

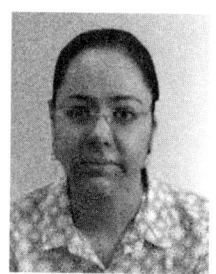

Jasmine Chawla
Assistant Professor
Amity Institute of Physiotherapy
Amity University
Noida, Uttar Pradesh

Preface

Orthopedics is a short subject in the final year MBBS and there is pressure to cover up the major subjects. Towards the end as the examination approaches, many students tend to skip the subject in the last due to sheer voluminous nature of the books available in the market today.

Many a times the questions which are repeatedly asked in the examination are not covered in the textbooks. So, even after great efforts the results are not as desired. The book has been developed keeping in mind the most important questions asked in the examination. Question bank has been taken from Delhi Univeristy, Baba Farid University of Health Sciences, Rajasthan University and Postgraduate Institute of Medical Sciences, Rohtak.

The text has been written in such a manner that it can be reproduced in the examination with ease. The book has been divided into familiar sections like general orthopedics, trauma and others. The division shall give readers an easy and comprehensive experience. The book shall relieve many students from the last moment examination stress.

The book shall provide concise, consolidated and trustworthy coverage of the subject of orthopedics. A large number of textbooks and journals has been referred before compiling this book. I would still accept the constructive criticism and fruitful suggestions.

Kavin Khatri

Contents

Chapter 1

General Orthopedics

Q1. Write a short note on fracture union.

(5, *BFUHS May 2016, 2, RJ,*
January 2016)

Or

Write a short note on bone healing.

(3, *DU*)

Ans: Definition: It is a complex sequence of events to restore injured bone to pre-fracture state.

Stages of fracture healing

The fracture usually passes through following stages of healing:

1. *Stage of hematoma*
   - There is collection of blood at the fracture site and hematoma formation.
   - This stage lasts for one to two days.

2. *Stage of granulation tissue formation*
   - Aseptic necrosis at the fracture margins.
   - The multipotent cells collected at the fracture site undergoes transformation into osteoblast, chondroblast and fibroblast.

3. *Stage of soft callus (cartilage) formation*
   - Granulation tissues mature into fibrocartilaginous mass which transforms into spongy soft bone.
   - This stage lasts for 2 to 4 weeks.

4. *Stage of hard callus (bone) formation*
   - The soft callus is replaced with hard callus.
   - The spongy bone is replaced with mature lamellar bone.

5. *Stage of remodeling*
   - Newly formed bone undergoes changes as per the stress and strains over the bone.
   - The extra callus formed is resorbed.
   - It takes around 3 to 6 months for complete process.

Types

a. *Primary bone or fracture healing*
   - Fracture heals without extensive callus formation.
   - The stage of cartilage formation is not there and direct endosteal formation is present.
   - Seen in cases when rigid fixation like plating is utilized.

b. *Secondary bone or fracture healing*
   - Fracture heals with extensive callus formation.
   - Seen in cases treated with cast or sometimes in interlocking nail fixation.

Factors affecting fracture union

a. *Local factors*
   - Soft issue interposition
   - Open fracture
   - Pathological fracture
   - Infection
   - Comminuted fracture
   - Vascular injury
   - High energy injury

b. *Systemic factors*
   - Age: Faster in young and slower in elderly
   - Systemic diseases like diabetes, malignancy, thyroid disorders delay fracture union.
   - Hormonal factors: Prolonged steroid intake, growth hormone deficiency

- Smoking
- Drugs like NSAIDs, phenytoin

Q2. Define dislocation and subluxation.
(1, RJ January 2011)

Ans: Dislocation: When there is no contact between articular surfaces and they are completely displaced.

Subluxation: When there is some contact between articular surfaces and they are partially displaced.

Q3. Name different types of splint and their uses.
(3, DU)

Ans: Splints are used to immobilize a particular part of body. The commonly used splints are

1. Wooden splints
2. Metallic splints
3. Plaster splints
4. Pneumatic/inflatable splints
5. Miscellaneous—newspapers, cardboards, etc.

Indications/uses of splint

- Temporary immobilization of sprains, fractures, and unreduced dislocations.
- Pain control
- Prevention of neurovascular injuries.

Contraindications

- Open fractures
- Suspected compartment syndrome
- Neurovascular compromise
- Reflex sympathetic dystrophy

Q4. Write a short note on basic method of treating fracture.
(5, RJ January 2016)

Ans: Treatment of fracture can be considered in three phases

- Phase I: Emergency care
- Phase II: Definitive care
- Phase III: Rehabilitation.

Phase I: Emergency care: At the site of accident, splinting is done to relieve pain, prevent movement, prevent damage to the skin, soft tissue and neurovascular structure, prevent complications like fat embolism and make patient's transportation easier.

In emergency department, provide basic life support, if patient is in shock.

- A quick evaluation of extent of injury.
- If any bleeding then stop it with pressure.
- Check splinting.
- Analgesics as per requirement.

Phase II: Definitive care: Three fundamental principles are used in case of fracture: (i) Reduction, (ii) immobilization, and (iii) preservation of functions.

  i. *Reduction*: Only displaced fractures are needed to be reduced. Reduction can be carried out by following methods
- Closed manipulation
- Continuous traction
- Open reduction

  ii. *Immobilization*
- It prevents displacement or angulation of fracture.
- Prevents movement that might interfere with the union.
- Relieves pain.

Following methods can be used for immobilization
- Strapping
- Sling
- Cast immobilization
- Functional bracing
- Splints and traction
- Operative methods—internal fixation or external fixation

iii. *Preservation of functions:* It essentially consists of muscle re-education exercises and instructions regarding mobilization of the limb.

Phase III: Rehabilitation: In this phase, the strengthening exercises, gait training, etc. are carried out so that patient returns to his/her original form.

Q5. Write a short note on epiphyseal injuries.

(*2, RJ January 2015, 3, DU*)

Ans: Epiphysis or growth plate is present at the end of long bones. It helps in growth of the bone. An injury involving the growth plate results in deformities due to irregular growth, and shortening.

Various classification methods are used to classify epiphyseal injuries. Salter-Harris classification is most commonly used classification system and is described below

Type I: There is break through the growth plate separating bone end from shaft.

Type II: There is break through part of bone at growth plate and through bone shaft.

Type III: The fracture line passes through growth plate and through bone end.

Type IV: The fracture break through bone shaft, growth plate and bone end.

Type V: There is compression of growth plate due to compression forces.

Salter-Harris classification

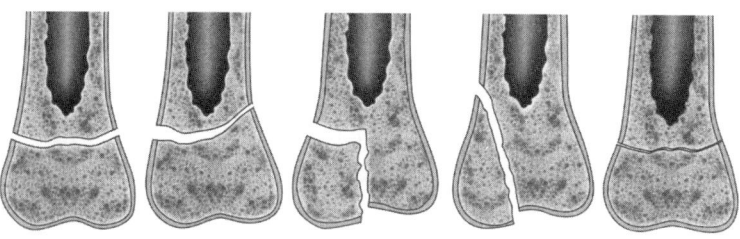

Type 1   Type 2   Type 3   Type 4   Type 5

Diagnosis: X-rays can be used to diagnose epiphyseal injuries. The opposite limb radiographs can be used in doubtful cases.

Treatment

- Reduction (closed or open) if needed with internal fixation depending upon the fracture pattern.

- Type V epiphyseal injuries are usually detected at later stages.

Chapter 2

Peripheral Nerve Injuries

Q1. Write a short note on ulnar nerve palsy.

(5, BFUHS November 2012,
May 2012, 3 DU)

Or

Write a short note on high ulnar nerve palsy. (3, DU)

Or

Write a short note on ulnar claw hand—pathology and management. (3, DU, 3, DU)

Ans: Ulnar nerve palsy leads to weakness in hand and loss of sensation over the medial aspect of hand.

Etiology

- Injury around elbow (supracondylar fracture, elbow dislocation)
- *Abnormal growth*: Tumor or cyst pressing over the nerve
- Leprosy
- Penetrating injuries around elbow and wrist.

Type

- *High ulnar nerve palsy*: Involvement of ulnar nerve above elbow joint
- *Low ulnar nerve palsy*: Involvement of ulnar nerve at or below elbow joint

Clinical features

High ulnar nerve palsy

- There is paralysis of all muscles supplied by the ulnar nerve.
- On palmar flexing wrist, the hand deviates towards the radial side. Due to paralysis of flexor carpi ulnaris, there is unopposed action of flexor carpi radialis which deviates the wrist towards radial (outer) side.
- There is wasting of hypothenar muscles.
- *Egawa's test*: The patient cannot move his middle finger sideways due to involvement of dorsal interossei. The dorsal interossei help in abduction of finger (mnemonic: DAB—dorsal abduction).
- *Card test*: The patient cannot hold card tightly between fingers due to involvement of palmar interossei. The palmar interossei helps in adduction of finger (mnemonic: PAD—palmar adduction).
- *Fromet sign*: The patient is asked to hold book between thumb and index finger. Due to involvement of adductor pollicis, he/she tries to hold the book with flexion at interphalangeal joint of thumb (action of flexor pollicis is supplied by median nerve).
- *Claw hand*: There is flexion at interphalangeal joints and extension at metacarpophalangeal joint. The common digital extensor contract to produce this deformity. It is limited to ring and little fingers.
- *Sensory loss*: There is loss of sensation over the anterior, medial and posterior aspects of medial one-third of hand. There is also loss of medial one and a half fingers.

Low ulnar nerve palsy: The presentation is similar to high ulnar nerve palsy, except following differences:

- There is no deviation at wrist on palmar flexion as flexor carpi ulnaris is spared.
- There is exaggerated ulnar clawing (also known as ulnar paradox) due to sparing of medial half of flexor

digitorum profundus. The unopposed contraction of both common digital extensors and flexors leads to exaggerated deformity.

- The sensory loss is limited to medial one and a half fingers (half of ring finger and little finger).

Diagnosis

Nerve conduction velocity: The part of the nerve proximal to the nerve is stimulated with electric current and conduction is assessed. In case of complete nerve injury there is complete loss of transmission and in compressive lesions the transmission (or conduction) is delayed.

Electromyography

- Helps in detecting the level of injury
- Differentiate between complete and incomplete injury
- Helps in assessing the recovery after nerve repair.

Treatment

Non-operative

- Support the limb with knuckle bender splint
- Range of motions exercises at wrist and small joints of hand to prevent contracture
- Extra care for limb due to loss of sensation.
- Drugs like methylcobalamin, pregabalin and pain killers
- Nerve muscle stimulation to prevent muscular atrophy

Operative

- Nerve repair in acute cases
- *Neurolysis:* The nerve is freed from surrounding fibrous tissue.
- *Tendon transfer:* When the surgery for nerve repair is delayed beyond one year, there is complete degeneration of neuromuscular junction and hence recovery is not possible.

The tendons commonly used for transfer are:

1. Single slip of flexor digitorum superficialis
2. Brachioradialis

3. Flexor carpi radialis
4. Palmaris longus

Q2. Write a short note on radial nerve palsy.

(5, BFUHS May 2009, 5,
RJ January 2011)

Or

Write a short note on lower radial nerve palsy.

(2, RJ Janauary 2013, 5,
RJ January 2009)

Or

Write a short note on wrist drop.   *(3, DU)*

Ans: Radial nerve palsy or involvement leads to weakness in extension at wrist and loss of sensation over the dorsal aspect of hand.

Etiology
- Fracture of shaft of humerus
- Improper use of axillary crutches
- Direct penetrating trauma over arm
- Post-surgery fixation of humerus fracture or after closed reduction of fracture.
- Sleeping in arm in abduction and pressure over the axilla
- Leprosy

Type
- *Very high radial nerve palsy*: Involvement of radial nerve injury above the spiral groove.
- *High radial nerve palsy*: Involvement of radial nerve injury between spiral groove and elbow.
- *Low radial nerve palsy*: Involvement of radial nerve injury below the elbow.

Clinical features
Very high radial nerve palsy
- Radial nerve supplies motor innervation to triceps, brachioradialis, supinator, the wrist, finger, and thumb extensors.

- There is paralysis of all the muscles supplied by radial nerve.
- Loss of extension at elbow, wrist and fingers
- Sensory loss: There is loss of sensation over the posterior and inferolateral aspect of arm, posterior forearm, dorsal aspect of wrist and hand.

High radial nerve palsy

- There is loss of extension at wrist and finger extension
- Sensory loss: dorsal aspect of wrist and hand.

Low radial nerve palsy

- There is loss of finger extension
- Sensory loss: Loss of sensation over the 1st dorsal web space.
- Below elbow joint, the radial nerve is divided into motor branch (posterior interosseous nerve) and sensory branch (superficial radial nerve). In case only motor branch is damaged, there is loss of finger extension only and no sensory loss.

Diagnosis

Nerve conduction velocity: The part of the nerve proximal to the nerve is stimulated with electric current and conduction is assessed. In case of complete nerve injury, there is complete loss of transmission and in compressive lesions, the transmission (or conduction) is delayed.

Electromyography

- It helps in detecting the level of injury
- To differentiate between complete and incomplete injury
- To assess the recovery after nerve repair

Treatment

Non-operative

- Support the limb with wrist drop splint
- Range of motion exercises at wrist and small joints of hand to prevent contracture.

- Extra care for limb due to loss of sensation.
- Drugs like methylcobalamin, pregabalin and pain killers.
- Nerve muscle stimulation to prevent muscular atrophy.

Operative
- Nerve repair in acute cases
- *Neurolysis*: The nerve is freed from surrounding fibrous tissue.
- *Tendon transfer*: One or multiple tendons (flexor carpi ulnaris, pronator teres, Flexor digitorum superficialis, palmaris longus) can be transferred from palmar aspect of forearm to dorsal side and extension at wrist and fingers can thus be achieved.

Q3. Write a short note on median nerve palsy.

(5, BFUHS May 2006, 5, BFUHS November 2011)

Or

Write a short note on pointing index finger test.

(3, DU)

Or

Enumerate the clinical tests you would perform to assess the function of median nerve. *(3, DU)*

Ans: Median nerve palsy or involvement leads to weakness in hand and loss of sensation over the lateral aspect of hand.

Etiology
- Direct penetrating injury
- Rheumatoid arthritis
- Diabetes
- Obesity
- Pregnancy
- Use of vibrating tool-like stone cutter

Clinical features
- There is paralysis of all the muscles supplied by median nerve

- Loss of flexion at metacarpophalangeal and inter-Pphalangeal joints of all the fingers (due to involvement of flexor digitorum profundus, flexor digitorum superficialis, flexor pollicis longus).
- Ape thumb deformity: In this deformity, the thumb is adducted and extended.
- Pointing index sign: On making fist, the index finger remains straight due to involvement of flexor digitorum superficialis and lateral half of flexor digitorum profundus in cases of median nerve involvement proximal to elbow.
- Wasting of thenar muscles
- Sensory loss: There is loss of sensation over the palmar aspect of lateral two-thirds of palm, thumb, index, middle and lateral half of ring fingers.

Diagnosis

- *Nerve conduction velocity*: The part of the nerve proximal to the nerve is stimulated with electric current and conduction is assessed. In case of complete nerve injury, there is complete loss of transmission and in compressive lesions, the transmission (or conduction) is delayed.
- *Electromyography*
  a. It helps in detecting the level of injury.
  b. To differentiate between complete and incomplete injury.
  c. To assess the recovery after nerve repair.

Treatment
Non-operative
- Support the limb with opponens splint
- Range of motion exercises at wrist and small joints of hand to prevent contracture
- Extra care for limb due to loss of sensation.
- Drugs like methylcobalamin, pregabalin and pain killers.

• Nerve muscle stimulation to prevent muscular atrophy.

Operative

• Nerve repair in acute cases
• Neurolysis: The nerve is freed from surrounding fibrous tissue
• Tendon transfer: The tendons used singly or in combination are as follows:
  a. Palmaris longus
  b. Extensor indices proprius
  c. Abductor digiti minimi

Q4. Write a short note on foot drop.

(*5, BFUHS November 2009, 1, RJ, January 2011*)

Ans: Foot drop is loss of extension at ankle and digits of foot due to injury to some fibres of sciatic nerve or deep peroneal nerve.

Etiology

• Injuries around hip joint such as posterior hip dislocation and acetabular fractures
• Injuries around knee joint such as knee dislocation and proximal tibia fractures
• Intramuscular injection in gluteal region
• Leprosy
• Lumbar disc prolapse
• Tight plaster application around knee joint
• Skeletal traction application around knee joint
• Direct penetrating trauma.

Clinical features

• There is inability to dorsiflex at ankle and digits of foot
• High steppage gait
• Wasting of muscles of leg

- Sensory loss: There is loss of sensation over the lateral aspect of leg and dorsum of foot.

Diagnosis

Nerve conduction velocity: The part of the nerve proximal to the nerve is stimulated with electric current and conduction is assessed. In case of complete nerve injury, there is complete loss of transmission and in compressive lesions, the transmission (or conduction) is delayed.

Electromyography

- It helps in detecting the level of injury
- To differentiate between complete and incomplete injury
- To assess the recovery after nerve repair.

Treatment

Non-operative

- Support the limb with foot drop splint
- Range of motion exercises at knee and small joints of feet to prevent contracture
- Extra care for limb due to loss of sensation.
- Drugs like methylcobalamin, pregabalin and pain killers
- Nerve muscle stimulation to prevent muscular atrophy.

Operative

- Nerve repair in acute cases
- *Neurolysis:* The nerve is freed from surrounding fibrous tissue
- *Tendon transfer*
    a. Tibialis posterior is transferred from posterior compartment to anterior compartment.
    b. Peroneus longus is another tendon used in foot drop
- Ankle arthrodesis: In neglected cases.

Q5. Discuss Seddon's classification of nerve injury.

(5, RJ January 2016)

Ans: Seddon classified localized injuries to peripheral nerves after study of large numbers of casualties during second World War.

He described injuries as

a. Neurapraxia

b. Axonotmesis

c. Neurotmesis

Neurapraxia

- It is focal nerve compression
- There is reversible conduction block without wallerian degeneration
- *Etiology:* Local ischemia
- *Histopathology:* There is focal demyelination of the axon sheath.
- Nerve conduction velocity shows complete conduction block and there are no fibrillation potentials.
- Prognosis is excellent. There is full recovery of the nerve.

Axonotmesis

- *Histopathology:* Axon and myelin sheath disruption leads to conduction block with wallerian degeneration.
- Nerve conduction velocity shows fibrillations and positive sharp waves on electromyography (EMG).
- *Prognosis:* Good. There is almost complete recovery of the involved nerve.

Neurotmesis

- *Histopathology:* Complete nerve division with disruption of endoneurium.
- Nerve conduction velocity shows fibrillations and positive sharp waves on EMG.

• Prognosis is variable. Surgical repair of the nerve is required.

Q6. Write a short note on Erb's palsy. (3, DU)

Ans: It is most common birth related neurapraxia.

Pathology

• There is involvement of nerve root C5 and C6.
• There is lesion of *axillary, musculocutaneous* and *suprascapular nerves.*
• In severely affected patients *deltoid, biceps, brachialis,* and *subscapular* are affected.

Clinical features

• The arm cannot be raised since deltoid and spinal muscles are paralyzed.
• Elbow flexion is weakened because of involvement of biceps and brachialis.
• After six months, there are contractures of muscles leading to internal rotation and adduction.

Investigations

X-ray: It can detect cervical rib which has high association with Erb's palsy.

EMG: It can differentiate between reversible *vs* irreversible nerve damage.

Treatment

• Majority of the cases recover on their own
• Range of motion exercises at shoulder to retain abduction and external rotation at shoulder.
• Nerve grafting
• Contracture release
• Tendon transfer

Q7. Write a short note on tardy ulnar nerve palsy. (3, DU)

Ans: Tardy ulnar nerve palsy is gradual involvement of the ulnar nerve due to various reasons.

Etiology

- Neglected non-union of lateral condyle humerus, malunited supracondylar humerus.
- Thickening of ligament or muscle passing through the course of nerve.
- Hormonal disorders like acromegaly, diabetes.

Symptoms

- Numbness along the lateral half of ring finger and little finger.
- Weakness of the hand grip
- There is worsening of the symptoms.

Diagnosis

- Nerve conduction velocity shows decrease in nerve conduction of ulnar nerve.
- Electromyography.

Treatment: Transposition of the ulnar nerve anteriorly across elbow from the usual position of posterior to medial epicondyle.

Chapter 3

Complications of Fracture

Q1. Write a short note on Sudeck's osteodystrophy.

(3, BFUHS May 2008, 5, BFUHS May 2016)

Or

Write a short note on clinical features of Sudeck's osteodystrophy. *(3, DU)*

Ans: Definition: Reflex sympathetic dystrophy (RSD) is characterized by group of symptoms like burning type pain, tenderness, and swelling of an extremity associated with sweating, warmth, flushing, discoloration, and shiny skin.

Etiopathogenesis: The exact mechanism of reflex sympathetic dystrophy is not fully understood. There are theories like neural dysfunction, inflammatory neuronal reaction, sympathetic system dysfunction which have been postulated.

The triggering factors postulated as follows:

• After upper limb surgery or injury

• Heart disease

• Stroke

• Degenerative disease of neck

• Nerve entrapment syndrome like carpal tunnel syndrome

Clinical features

The symptomatology in RSD depends upon the stage of presentation:

- *Acute stage* (three to six months): There is burning, flushing, sweating, swelling, pain out of proportion to injury and tenderness.
- *Dystrophic stage* (six months to one year): Changes in skin appear like thickening along with joint stiffness.
- *Atrophic stage* (after one year): There are fixed joint contractures and significant loss of subcutaneous fat. The radiographs show marked osteoporosis.

Diagnosis

- *X-ray* shows features of osteoporosis
- *MRI* shows soft tissue edema and patchy bone marrow edema.
- *Bone scan:* It shows increased uptake on all three phases. There is increased activity around joints.

Treatment

- Cool and moist applications to the affected areas.
- Range of motion exercises to prevent joint contractures.
- Medicine for pain relief and inflammation.
- Gradual exercise can help prevent contractures.
- NSAIDs, high dose of steroids, pregabalin and nifedipine have been tried with varied success.
- Nerve root block like stellate ganglion block
- Surgical sympathectomy
- Intrathecal pumps: Putting pain medication pumps in spinal canal.

Q2. Write a short note on open fractures.

(5, BFUHS, November 2013, 5, RJ January 2012)

Or

Write a short note on open fractures—definition, classification and management. *(3, DU)*

Ans: Open fracture or compound fracture in which there is break in the skin continuity with bony injury. Due to contamination of fracture site, there are high chances of complications like infection and non-union.

Etiology

- High energy trauma such as a gunshot or motor vehicle accident.
- Rarely low energy trauma such as fall at home in elderly population.

Classification: Gustilo-Anderson classification is used to classify the open fracture as follows:

Type I: When wound size is less than one centimeter and wound bed is clean with minimal contamination.

Type II: When wound size is between 1 to 10 cm with moderate soft tissue injury.

Type IIIA: When wound size is greater than 10 cm, high grade soft tissue injury requiring wound coverage. It includes segmental and severely comminuted fractures.

Type IIIB: When there is extensive periosteal stripping and requires free soft tissue transfer.

Type IIIC: Open fracture associated with vascular injury.

Treatment

- *Debridement and irrigation*: The wound is cleared of foreign and contaminated material. Wound is washed with several liters of saline. The wound is cleared of all the devitalized tissue. The debridement should preferably be carried out within six hours of injury.

- *Antibiotic therapy*: For type I and type II open fractures, first generation cephalosporins are enough. For type III open fractures, metronidazole or penicillin may be added to cover the anaerobes. Anti-tetanus prophylaxis is given especially in type III wounds.

- *Fracture stabilization*: The fractures are stabilized with external fixator mainly. However, depending upon the wound condition, the decision to fix the fracture with nail or plate is taken. The cleaner wound can be primarily debrided and fixed in single sitting.

- *Amputation*: Amputation or removal of part of the limb is considered in cases of extensive wound contamination, soft tissue coverage not possible or life-threatening infection.

Complications
- Non-union
- Chronic pain syndrome
- Osteomyelitis

Q3. Write a short note on malunion (5, *BFUHS May 2007*)

Ans: Definition: Malunited fracture is one in which bony fragments are healed in malalignment.

Etiology
1. Malreduction
2. Inadequate immobilization during healing
3. Missed injury
4. Inadequate reduction in surgery
5. Inappropriate treatment chosen at first instance (like fracture requiring operation managed with non-operative methods)

Common sites of malunion: Fracture of distal end of radius and supracondylar humerus.

Clinical features
- Deformity of the limb
  - Stiffness may be associated to the adjoining joints
  - Muscular wasting
  - Loss of functionality

Implications of malunion
- Malunion leads to poor alignment of the limb and consequently puts uneven pressure on joints leading to early joint destruction.
- There is shortening of the limb
- Restriction of movements at adjoining joints.

Diagnosis

X-ray: Anteroposterior and lateral view of the involved limb shows malalignment.

Treatment

Non-operative: It can be considered in following circumstances:

a. Children with remaining growth potential have ability to remodel deformity.

b. Deformity up to 5° in coronal or sagittal plane gets corrected with remodeling but malrotation does not correct.

c. Some bones, like clavicle, unite in malunion but there is no functional disability so no operation is required.

d. Angular deformity in the plane of movement of adjoining joints remodels, e.g. anterior angulation in tibia.

e. Fractures in the metaphyseal region.

Operative

• Corrective osteotomy (surgically breaking the bone again) with plate or nail application.

• Ilizarov's technique for gradual correction of the deformity. It is used in long-standing cases to avoid neurovascular injury.

• Excision of the bony fragment impinging upon the skin.

Q4. Describe the clinicoradiological signs of myositis ossificans and its management.

(10, BFUHS, November 2006)

Or

Write a short note on myositis ossificans.

(5, BFUHS May 2013,5, BFUHS May 2016)

Ans: Definition: It is a reactive process in which there is well circumscribed proliferation of fibroblasts, bone or cartilage within muscle mass.

Incidence

• Most common in active young males.

• It is commonly seen in brachialis, deltoid and gluteal muscles.

- Aggressive massage following injury around elbow joint is the most common presenting feature.

Etiology

- Genetic predisposition has been proposed.
- Direct trauma has been implicated.
- Intramuscular hematoma is a predisposing factor.

Histopathology

- Center of lesion shows irregular mass of immature fibroblasts with or without cartilage and no atypical cells.
- Peripheral lesion shows mature trabeculae of lamellar and woven bone.

Clinical features

Acute stage: Pain, swelling, tenderness and restriction of movement at the joint.

Late stage: Bony swelling with mechanical block to movement. There is no pain at this stage.

Diagnosis

Blood test

- *Creatine kinase*: It is elevated and higher levels correlate with widespread involvement.
- *C-reactive protein*: Elevated in acute stage.
- *Serum alkaline phosphatase*: May be elevated in few cases.

Radiograph: In acute stage there is patchy, flocculent appearance on X-rays. In late stage, there is peripheral calcification with central radiolucent area.

CT scan: It shows egg shell appearance in mature or late stage

MRI: There is rim enhancement in early stages and it also helps in surgical planning.

Bone scan: There is increased uptake on three-phase bone scan.

Treatment

Non-operative

- Rest and range of motion exercises at the adjacent joints.
- Avoid passive stretching
- Extracorporeal shock wave therapy: It can reduce the pain and helps in increasing the range of motion.

Operative

- The lesion is radiographically monitored till its maturity. It takes around 6 to 12 months for it to mature fully.
- The lesion is excised after maturity as there are high chances of recurrence on its removal before maturity.

Prophylaxis

- *Drug prophylaxis*
  a. NSAIDs like indomethacin given in dosage of 75 mg/day for 3 weeks.
  b. Rofecoxib decreases the risk of ossificans.
  c. Bisphosphonates decrease the incidence of ossificans.
- *Radiation therapy:* It is helpful in decreasing the chances of ossification in high risk cases.

Q5. Describe in detail about the etiopathogenesis and management of non-union of fractures.

(10, BFUHS May 2008, 10, BFUHS November 2007)

Or

Describe in detail the causes of non-union and its management. *(10, BFUHS November 2009)*

Or

Write a short note on non-union.

(5, BFUHS May 2018, 3, BFUHS May 2014, 1, RJ January 2011, 3, DU, 3, DU)

Or

Write a short note on clinical and radiological features of non-union. (5, BFUHS May 2015)

Or

Write a short note on causes of non-union. (3, DU)

Ans: Definition: According to FDA (food and drug administration, USA) non-union is "established when a minimum of 9 months has elapsed since injury and the fracture shows no visible progressive signs of healing for 3 months".

Etiology

Local factors
- Open fractures
- Infection
- Soft interposition
- Inadequate immobilization
- Avascular necrosis
- Distraction at the fracture site
- Segmental fracture

Systemic factors
- Smoking
- Prolonged steroid intake
- NSAIDs
- Metabolic disorders

Classification
1. *Hypervascular or hypertrophic non-union*: It is rich in callus and high vascularity at the bony ends.
2. *Avascular or atrophic non-union*: Callus is absent and poor blood supply.
3. *Oligotrophic non-union*: Callus is absent however fracture ends are vascular.
4. *Comminuted non-union*: It is characterized by one or two necrotic intermediate fragments.
5. *Defect non-union*: There is loss of bony fragment between the two segments.

6. *Infected non-union*: Infection at the fracture margins leads to osteomyelitis and non-union.

Diagnosis

X-ray: It shows the sclerotic fracture margins, no crossing trabaculae across the fracture site.

Bone scan: Helps in detecting the vascularity of the fracture margins.

Treatment: The principle in treatment is to identify the reason for non-union and treat the same.

Non-operative

• Low intensity ultrasound: It stimulates bone healing
• Electromagnetic stimulation across fracture site
• Bone morphogenic proteins

Operative

Hypertrophic non-union: Internal fixation is only required to achieve union

Avascular or atrophic non-union: Freshening of bone margins along with internal fixation and bone grafting.

Comminuted non-union: Removal of the necrotic fragment and internal fixation with bone grafting.

Defect non-union: Filling of defect with bone grafting or bone transport with ilizarov technique.

Infected non-union: Staged treatment is preferred. In first stage, infected or devitalized tissue is removed and in second stage bone transport is carried out.

Q6. Write a short note on clinical features of acute compartment syndrome.

(5, BFUHS May 2015, 2.5, RJ 2015, 2, RJ January 2013, 5, RJ January 2011)

Or

Write a short note on pathophysiology of compartment syndrome.   *(5, BFUHS May 2017)*

Or

Write a short note on compartment syndrome.

(3, DU, 3, DU, 3, DU)

Ans: Definition: It is elevation of interstitial pressure in closed osteofascial compartment resulting in microvascular compromise.

Etiology

- Fracture of both bones—forearm and leg
- Tight plaster application
- Damage to artery
- Burn
- Anticoagulant
- Patients with altered consciousness.

Pathophysiology

Increased osteofascial compartment pressure either due to external compression or internal edema secondary to injury leads to decrease in venous return leading to further edema and increase in compartmental pressure. The raised compartmental pressure leads to tissue necrosis and this viscous cycle continues.

Common sites of compartment syndrome

1. Deep posterior compartment of leg
2. Foot
3. Forearm
4. Hand

Clinical features: The presentation of compartment can be described in 5 Ps:

- Pain: Severe pain disproportionate to injury
- Paresthesia
- Pallor
- Pulselessness
- Paralysis of the involved muscles

Diagnosis: It is mainly clinical. The clinical features are the major diagnostic criteria. Intracompartmental pressure can be measured with hand held manometers. Intracompartmental pressure greater than 30 mm Hg is suggests compartment syndrome.

Treatment
- Fasciotomy is performed as an emergency procedure
- Fracture is reduced
- Kidneys are protected with intravenous fluids and urine output is maintained with help of diuretics if required.

Q7. Write a short note on gas gangrene.

(1, RJ January 2011, 1, RJ January 2009)

Ans: Definition: It is infection of muscle tissue by toxin producing clostridia.

Risk factors: Various risk factors for gas gangrene are:
- Postoperative:
  – Bile duct surgery
  – Bowel perforation
- Post-traumatic:
  – Crush injury
  – Gunshot wound
  – Intravenous drug abuse
- Spontaneous:
  – Colon cancer
  – Neutropenia

Pathophysiology
- Gas gangrene is caused by an anaerobic, gram-positive, spore-forming bacillus of the genus Clostridium. *C. perfringens* is the most common etiologic agent that causes gas gangrene.
- Alpha toxin produced by clostridia induces necrosis by causing the rapid loss of intracellular potassium and depletion of adenosine triphosphate (ATP).
- Systemically, exotoxins may cause severe hemolysis. Hemoglobin level decreases and leads to hypotension and acute tubular necrosis.

Clinical features

Symptoms

• Sudden increase in pain out of proportion to injury due to thrombotic occlusion of large vessels.

• Felling of uneasiness.

Signs

• Tachycardia
• Sweet smelling odor
• Swelling, edema, discoloration and ecchymosis
• Blebs and hemorrhagic bullae
• Purulent discharge
• Altered mental status
• Purulent discharge

Investigations

• *Blood tests*: Elevated white blood cells, lactate dehydrogenase, metabolic acidosis.

• *Histopathology*: Gram staining reveals gram-positive bacteria and lack of inflammatory response.

• *Blood culture*: It can isolate clostridia species

Treatment

Non-operative

• Intravenous penicillin and clindamycin
• Erythromycin and tetracycline are other alternatives
• Hyperbaric oxygen

Operative

Radical surgical debridement with fasciotomies.

Q8. Write a short note on complications of open fracture of both bone leg. *(5, RJ January 2011)*

Ans: The complications of open fracture of both bones leg can be classified as:

a. Early complications
b. Late complications

Early complications

1. *Vascular injury*: Fractures of the proximal half of the tibia may damage the popliteal artery. This is an

emergency of the first order, requiring exploration and repair. Damage to one of the two major tibial vessels may also occur.

2. *Compartment syndrome*: The combination of tissue edema and bleeding causes swelling in the muscle compartments and this may precipitate ischemia. Additional risk factors are proximal tibial fractures, severe crush injury, a long ischemic period before revascularization (in type IIIC open fractures), a long delay to treatment, hemorrhagic shock, difficult and prolonged operation and a fracture fixed in distraction. The diagnosis can be confirmed by measuring the compartment pressures in the leg. A differential pressure (ΔP) the difference between diastolic pressure and compartment pressure of less than 30 mm Hg (4.00 kPA) is regarded as critical and an indication for compartment decompression.

3. *Fasciotomy and decompression*: Once the diagnosis is made, decompression should be carried out with the minimum delay. This is best and most safely accomplished through two incisions; one anterolateral and one posteromedial.

4. Infection even a small perforation should be treated with respect and debridement carried out before the wound is closed. If the diagnosis is suspected, wound swabs and blood samples should be taken and antibiotic treatment started forthwith, using a 'best guess' intravenous preparation; once the laboratory results are obtained, a more suitable antibiotic may be substituted.

Late complications

1. *Malunion*: Slight shortening (up to 1.5 cm) is usually of a little consequence, but rotation and angulation deformity, apart from being unsightly, can be disabling because the knee and ankle no longer move in the same plane. Varus or valgus angulation will alter the axis of loading through the knee or ankle, causing increased stress in some part of the joint. Late

deformity, if marked, should be corrected by tibial osteotomy.

2. *Delayed union*: High energy fractures are slow to unite and liable to non-union or fatigue failure if a nail has been used. If there is a failure of union to progress on X-ray by 6 months, secondary intervention should be considered. The first nail is removed, the canal reamed and a larger nail reinserted. If the fibula has united before the tibia, it should be osteotomized so as to allow better apposition and compression of the tibial fragments.

3. *Non-union*: This may follow bone loss or deep infection, but a common cause is faulty treatment.

4. *Joint stiffness*: Prolonged cast immobilization is liable to cause stiffness of the ankle and foot, which may persist for 12 months or longer in spite of active exercises. This can be avoided by changing to a functional brace as soon as it is safe to do so, usually by 4–6 weeks.

5. *Osteoporosis*: Axial loading of the tibia is important and weight-bearing should be re-established as soon as possible.

6. *Regional complex pain syndrome*: With distal third fractures, this is not uncommon. Exercises should be encouraged throughout the period of treatment.

Q9. Write a short note on crush syndrome. *(3, DU)*

Ans: Crush syndrome is a consequence of:
- Prolonged continuous pressure on the limb
- Prolonged use of a pneumatic anti-shock garment.

Pathophysiology
- The crushed limb is underperfused and myonecrosis follows, leading to the release of toxic metabolites when the limb is freed and so generating a reperfusion injury.
- Reactive oxygen metabolites create further tissue injury. Membrane damage and capillary fluid reabsorption failure result in swelling that may lead

to a compartment syndrome, thus creating more tissue damage from escalating ischemia.

- Tissue necrosis also causes systemic problems such as renal failure from free myoglobin, which is precipitated in the renal glomeruli. Myonecrosis may cause a metabolic acidosis with hyperkalemia and hypocalcemia.

Clinical features
The compromised limb is pulseless and becomes red, swollen and blistered; sensation and muscle power may be lost.

Investigation
- Serum creatine phosphokinase (CPK) levels
- Urine myoglobin levels

Treatment

- Fluid is administered to correct hypovolemia to prevent renal shutdown and for clearance of myoglobin.
- Urine is alkalinization of urine with bicarbonate and acetazolamide.
- Mannitol infusion also limits tissue injury ischemia and reperfusion of organs.
- Potassium chloride diuretic drug decreases intra-cellular sodium concentration and inhibits sodium hydrogen and sodium calcium exchange.
- Intravenous calcium is only indicated in cases of hyperkalemic arrhythmia.

Chapter 4

Upper Limb Injuries

Q1. Describe mode of injury, complications and management of supracondylar fracture of humerus.

(15, BFUHS May 2006)

Or

Write a short note on complications of supracondylar fracture humerus. *(5, BFUHS November 2017)*

Or

Write a short note on supracondylar fracture of humerus. *(5, BFUHS May 2009)*

Or

Describe clinical features, treatment and complications of supracondylar fracture of humerus in children.

(10, BFUHS May 2014)

Or

Management of supracondylar fracture in children and enumerate its complications.

(10, BFUHS May 2015)

Or

Describe supracondylar humerus in children, its classification, clinical features, treatment and its complications. *(10, RJ January 2015)*

Or

Write a short note on Volksmann's ischemic contracture.

*(5, RJ, January 2011, 5,
RJ, January 2009, 3, DU)*

Ans: It is one of the most common and serious fractures encountered in childhood.

Mode or mechanism of injury and types:

1. *Extension type (more common)*: Fall on outstretched hand and elbow goes into extension resulting in fracture. The distal fragment is extended or tilted backwards.

2. *Flexion type*: Fall on flexed or bent elbow. The distal fragment here is tilted forwards or flexed.

Clinical features

• *Symptom:* Pain and swelling around the elbow. There is inability to move at elbow.

• *Signs*
  – Tenderness
  – S-shaped deformity of arm
  – The three-point bony relationship is maintained, i.e. the distance between medial epicondyle (one point), lateral epicondyle (another point) and olecranon (third point) is maintained.
  – The arm is shortened due to fracture
  – The vessels distal to fracture (radial and ulnar artery) should be palpated as sometimes the fracture may compress upon the brachial artery.
  – The integrity of nerves (median, ulnar and radial) should be checked by asking the patient to extend and flex at wrist along with sensory loss at the various nerves.

Management

Radiography: The anteroposterior and lateral view X-ray of the elbow helps in making the diagnosis. The distal fragment can be seen displaced on X-ray in following directions:

1. Posterior or backward tilt
2. Posterior or backward shift
3. Medial tilt
4. Medial or lateral shift
5. Internal rotation

Treatment

1. *Undisplaced fracture*: It requires immobilization in a plaster of Paris (POP) back slab.
2. *Displaced fracture*: It can be treated with:
   a. Closed reduction and POP back slab application
   b. Open reduction and internal fixation with Kirschner's wire.
   c. In case there is accompanying vessel injury, open reduction and internal fixation with Kirschner's wire and exploration of vessel.

Complications

Early complications

- Vascular injury (injury to brachial artery)
- Neurological injury (injury to median, radial and ulnar nerve)
- Compartment syndrome

Late complications

- Malunion
- Volksmann's ischemic contracture
- Myositis ossificans
- *Vascular injury*: The distal fragment sometimes presses upon the brachial artery and can present as vascular injury which may vary from intimal damage, vascular spasm and complete disruption of artery. The complete disruption of vessel can lead to dry gangrene.

  Diagnosis: Presentation is absence of palpable distal pulses.

  Treatment: Immediate exploration of brachial artery and fixation of fracture with Kirschner's wire. In case of complete disruption of brachial artery vascular repair is required.

- *Neurological injury*: The nerves involved in supracondylar fracture are median, radial and ulnar nerves. Majority of the times it is neurapraxia and requires no treatment. Surgical management is required if nerve function does not return after 2 months of injury.

• *Compartment syndrome*

Etiology: There is hematoma formation at the fracture site which compresses upon the venous return leading to increase in compartment pressure. The increased compartment pressure further leads to compromised venous return. So, this is a viscous cycle.

Diagnosis: It can be diagnosed clinically with features like pain, pallor, pulselessness, puffiness or swelling, paralysis and paresthesia (6 Ps). There are instruments like wick catheter which can measure the pressure.

Prevention: Limb elevation can increase the venous return hence chances of compartment syndrome are decreased.

Treatment
 – Fasciotomy at elbow and forearm can release the pressure.
 – Stabilization of fracture with Kirschner's wire.

• *Malunion:* It is the most common complication of the supracondylar humerus.

Etiology: It is due to union of fracture fragments in displaced position either initially at the time of injury or subsequently in plaster.

Types: The malunion can present as cubitus varus or valgus. Cubitus varus is the commoner among two. Cubitus varus is due to medial displacement and rotation of the distal fragment.

Clinical features: It is cosmetic deformity and there is no functional limitation in terms of movement at elbow joint.

Treatment

- Reassure the parents that it is a cosmetic deformity.
- Lateral closing wedge osteotomy
- Medial opening wedge osteotomy
- Dome osteotomy

• *Volkmann's ischemic contracture*

Etiology: It is due to prolonged ischemia of the forearm muscles leading to necrosis and fibrous tissue formation which undergoes contracture.

Clinical features

- There is peculiar deformity of hand in which flexion at wrist leads to extension at metacarpophalangeal joint and interphalangeal joint. The extension at wrist leads to flexion at metacarpophalangeal joint and interphalangeal joint.
- There is marked atrophy of muscles of forearm
- There is varied loss of sensation over the hand and forearm.
- There is atrophy of skin, nails and hair.

Grades

- *Mild:* Only flexor digitorum profundus and flexor hallucis longus is involved.
- *Moderate:* All the flexor muscles are involved
- *Severe:* Muscles of extensor group are also involved in addition to flexor group of muscles. There is also sensory loss.

Treatment

Mild grade: Splinting and range of motion exercises at joints of hand and wrist.

Moderate grade

- Excision of dead fibrotic tissue
- Release of flexor muscles from common flexor origin at medial epicondyle (maxpage operation)

Severe grade
- Wrist arthrodesis
- Proximal row carpectomy
- Shortening of bones of forearm
- *Myositis ossificans:* Read from question number 4, in Chapter 3.

Q2. Write a short note on dislocation of elbow.

(5, *BFUHS May 2006*)

Ans: It is the second most common dislocated joint after shoulder joint.

Mode or mechanism of injury: Fall on outstretched hand.

Types: According to the position of olecranon with respect to distal humerus it is classified as anterior or posterior.

Clinical features

- Pain and swelling over the elbow in flexed position in flexion type of dislocation.
- Prominence of olecranon
- The three-point bony relationship is disturbed.
- There may be associated fractures of medial epicondyle of humerus, radial head, distal humerus or coronoid.
- There may be associated injuries to the nerves like median, ulnar or radial.

Diagnosis: The anteroposterior and lateral radiographs of elbow can diagnose it.

Treatment

- Closed reduction with elbow in flexion and traction is given in the line of deformity. Subsequently plaster of Paris slab is given for 3 weeks.
- Open reduction and reconstruction of ligaments of elbow is done in cases of unstable reduction and old neglected cases.
- Open reduction and treatment of associated fractures.

Q3. Describe recurrent dislocation of shoulder.

(10, BFUHS November 2006)

Ans: Repeated dislocations at the shoulder joint is termed recurrent dislocation. Usually more than episodes of dislocation at the shoulder joint is termed a case of recurrent dislocation.

Types

- Anterior
- Posterior
- Inferior

Structural changes due to recurrent dislocation

- *Bankart lesion:* There is tear of fibrocartilaginous labrum along with periosteum and anterior capsule.
- *Hill-Sachs lesion:* There is defect over the postero-lateral aspect of the humeral head.
- There is stretching of the surrounding ligaments of the shoulder joint.
- There are bony and labral erosions due to repeated dislocation of the shoulder.

Clinical features

Symptoms: History of repeated dislocation of shoulder.

Signs

Wasting of deltoid muscle.

Tests for anterior instability

1. *Jobe's apprehension test:* Patient resists external rotation at the shoulder due to fear of shoulder dislocation.
2. *Anterior drawer test:* The head be translated anteriorly up to varying degree depending upon the degree of laxity.

Test for posterior instability

1. *Jobe's posterior apprehension test:* Patient resists internal rotation at the shoulder due to fear of shoulder dislocation.

2. *Posterior drawer test*: The head be translated posteriorly up to varying degree depending upon the degree of laxity.

Test for inferior instability

- *Sulcus sign*: On pulling down the arm, interval is seen between humeral head and acromion.

Diagnosis

Radiographs

- Anteroposterior and axillary views of shoulder can detect the shoulder dislocation.
- Special X-rays like west point view and stryker notch view can detect lesion like Hill-Sachs.

CT scan: It can quantify the bony defects in recurrent shoulder dislocation.

MRI: It can detect labral lesions, capsular laxity in addition to bony defects.

Treatment

Non-operative: Patients with generalized laxity of ligaments (those suffering from Marfan's syndrome, Ehlers-Danlos syndrome) are not benefited from surgery and are prescribed shoulder strengthening exercises.

Operative

1. Arthroscopic bankart repair: The bankart lesion is repaired though arthroscopic or keyhole surgery.
2. Open bankart repair
3. Puttiplatt operation: The subscapularis tendon is cut and overlapped (double breasted) so that the anterior structures are tightened and hence dislocation is prevented.
4. Latarjet procedure: Whenever there is large bony defects it requires reconstruction of glenoid with a piece of bone-like coracoid.

Q4. Describe in detail the clinical features, complications and management of shoulder dislocation.

(10, BFUHS November 2010)

Or
Write a short note on anterior dislocation of shoulder.
(5, BFUHS May 2012, 5,
BFUHS November 2012, 3, DU, 3, DU)

Ans: Shoulder joint is the most commonly dislocated joint of body.

Mode or mechanism of injury

• Fall on outstretched hand in abduction, external rotation and abduction.

• Direct trauma

Types

1. Anterior (most common)
2. Posterior
3. Inferior: Mostly seen after episodes of epilepsy.

Clinical features

Symptoms

• Pain and swelling around the shoulder joint
• Inability to move at the shoulder joint.

Signs

• Patient keeps his/her arm abducted supported with other hand.

• There is loss of contour of the shoulder

• Fullness in subclavicular region (anterior dislocation), posteriorly around shoulder (posterior dislocation) or in axilla (inferior dislocation).

• *Dugas test*: Inability to touch opposite shoulder with hand.

• *Callaway sign:* There is increase in girth of axilla as compared to normal side.

• *Hamilton ruler test:* In dislocated shoulder, on keeping a straight ruler over the lateral aspect of arm, it touches the acromion and lateral epicondyle simultaneously however in normal shoulder it is not possible.

Diagnosis

Radiography: Anteroposterior and axillary view radiographs can diagnose the dislocation.

CT scan is helpful in cases of posterior dislocation as it might be missed on anteroposterior view of shoulder radiograph.

Treatment

Non-operative: Majority of the shoulder dislocations can be reduced under general anesthesia with Kocher's maneuver, Hippocrates' method or Stimson's technique.

- *Kocher's maneuver:* The surgeon pulls the arm in line of deformity (Traction) with elbow in flexion, then Externally rotates the arm and Adduct the limb (mnemonic is TEA—traction external rotation and adduction). The assistant gives countertraction through a sheet passed across axilla.

- *Hippocrates method:* The surgeon put his foot in axilla and then pulls the arm in line of deformity.

- *Stimson's technique (used in posterior shoulder dislocation):* The patient is put in prone position and a weight of approximately 5 pounds is tied over the wrist and limb is hanged over the edge of table.

Operative: Open reduction is carried out in selected cases:
- Neglected shoulder dislocation
- Soft tissue interposition
- Associated fracture of head or neck of humerus.

Complications

- Axillary nerve injury
- Recurrent dislocation
- Brachial plexus injury
- Rotator cuff injury
- Associated fracture of greater tuberosity and neck of humerus
- Stiffness.

Q5. Write a short note on fracture clavicle.

(5, BFUHS, May 2007, 2, RJ January 2012)

Ans: It is one of the most common injuries across all population.

Mode/mechanism of injury

• Fall on outstretched hand

• Direct trauma

Displacement of fragments: Fracture clavicle generally occurs in the middle leading to formation of medial and lateral fragments. The medial fragment is displaced upwards due to pull of sternocleidomastoid and lateral fragment is pulled down by the weight of arm.

Clinical features

• *Symptoms:* Pain and swelling in the shoulder region.

• *Signs*

– Tenderness

– Crepitus can be elicited by moving the fragments.

– The vessels distal to fracture (brachial, radial and ulnar artery) should be palpated as sometimes the fracture may compress upon the subclavian artery.

– The integrity of nerves (median, ulnar and radial) should be checked by asking the patient to extend and flex at wrist along with sensory loss at the various nerves.

Diagnosis: Anteroposterior radiograph of shoulder can detect the fracture and its displacements.

Treatment

Non-operative: Majority of the clavicular fractures can be managed conservatively with help of clavicular brace or figure of "8" bandage and elbow pouch.

Operative

• Indications for operative intervention:

– Fracture of lateral end of clavicle

– Open fracture

– Both sides clavicle fracture

– Injury to the neurovascular bundle

- Operative options:
  - Closed reduction and fixation with flexible nails
  - Open reduction and fixation with plating

Complications

- Malunion
- Non-union
- Brachial plexus injury
- Injury to subclavian vessels
- Injury to apical lobe of lung

Q6. Write a short note on Colles' fracture

(5, BFUHS May 2008, 1,
RJ January 2011, 3,
DU, 3, DU, 3, DU, 3, DU)

Or

Define Colles' fracture. Discuss the mechanism of injury, sign and symptom, diagnosis and treatment of Colles' fracture. *(10, RJ January 2016)*

Ans: It is the fracture involving distal end of radius within 2 cm of distal radioulnar joint. It is one of the commonest fractures in osteoporotic females.

Mechanism or mode of injury: Fall on outstretched hand with wrist in dorsiflexion.

Clinical features

Symptoms

Pain and swelling around the wrist joint.

Signs

- Tenderness
- Dinner fork deformity
- Neurovascular assessment is carried out especially median nerve involvement.

Diagnosis: Anteroposterior and lateral radiographs of wrist joint show fracture of distal end of radius and displacement. The pattern of displacement of distal radius is as follows:

1. Dorsal tilt
2. Dorsal displacement
3. Lateral tilt
4. Lateral displacement
5. Impaction
6. Supination

Treatment

- *Non-operative*: Majority of the cases can be managed with closed reduction and plaster of Paris cast application.
- *Operative*
  - *Indications*
    1. Marked displacement
    2. Articular involvement
    3. Bilateral fracture
    4. Open fracture
    5. Secondary loss of reduction after closed reduction
  - *Operative options*
    a. Closed reduction and Kirschner's wire fixation
    b. Open reduction and internal fixation with plating
    c. External fixator application

Q7. Complications of Colles' fracture.

(5, BFUHS November 2010, 1, RJ January 2009)

Ans: Colles' fracture is the fracture involving distal end of radius within 2 cm of distal radioulnar joint. The complications encountered with Colles' fracture are as follows:

a. **Stiffness:** It is most commonly seen in patients treated with cast application. With regular movements stiffness at the wrist joint can be treated in majority of the cases.

b. **Compressive neuropathies:** The early complication is seen generally within first two weeks of injury.

Median nerve is the most common nerve involved in compressive neuropathy. The area affected by median nerve should be assessed after closed reduction of Colles' fracture.

c. **Arthritis of wrist joint:** It is another complication presenting with weakness of hand grip and pain in wrist on movement. Wrist splinting and pain killers help to overcome the condition.

d. **Loss reduction after reduction:** Sometimes there is loss of reduction after closed reduction on follow-up X-rays. It may require repeat reduction or sometimes open reduction and internal fixation.

e. **Sympathetic dystrophy:** Patients present with pain, swelling, discoloration of hand (redness or pallor), abnormal skin temperature relative to other hand and restricted movements of wrist and hand with reduced full fist grip.

Q8. Write a short note on fracture scaphoid.

(5, BFUHS November 2009, 5, BFUHS November 2010, 3, DU)

Or

Discuss management of fracture scaphoid.

(10, BFUHS November 2013)

Ans: It is the most common carpal bone injury. Majority of the times young adults are involved.

Blood supply of scaphoid: Scaphoid receives its blood supply from a vessel arising from radial artery. The vessel enters the scaphoid through distal pole and passes through the waist to supply the proximal pole. In case of fracture of scaphoid there is disruption, this blood supply leading to the complications like avascular necrosis.

Mechanism or mode of injury: Fall on outstretched hand leading to extension at wrist.

Clinical features

Symptoms: Pain and swelling in the anatomical snuff box.

Signs

Watson's test: Keeping the forearm pronated, the wrist is deviated from a position of ulnar deviation and extension to radial deviation and flexion at wrist. The presence of pain on movement is indicative of a fracture.

Management

Radiography: Anteroposterior and lateral radiographs of the wrist along with oblique views of the wrist help in diagnosing the fracture.

CT scan: It can detect the fracture with better sensitivity than X-rays and help in surgical planning.

MRI scan: It is highly sensitive investigation and can detect undisplaced fractures missed on other diagnostic modalities. It is also useful in assessing the vascularity of the fragments.

Bone scan: It can detect undisplaced fracture after 2 to 3 days after injury. There is increased uptake of radioactive material at the fracture site.

Treatment

Undisplaced fracture: Scaphoid cast (below elbow cast in hand holding position) is applied for 12 weeks. In case a person complains of pain in anatomical snuffbox. The scaphoid cast is applied for 2 weeks and then repeat X-rays are done to look for signs of fracture as many times as on initial presentation the fracture is missed on plain radiographs.

Displaced fracture: Closed or open reduction and internal fixation with Herbert screws (headless screws).

Complications

1. Delayed union
2. Non-union
3. Avascular necrosis
4. Secondary osteoarthritis of wrist

Q9. Write a short note on non-union scaphoid.

(*5, BFUHS May 2012, 5, BFUHS November 2012*)

Ans: Scaphoid is susceptible to poor healing because of its limited blood supply.

Blood supply of scaphoid: Same as in above question

Mechanism of injury: Same as above

Clinical features

Signs: Same as above

Symptoms: Same as above

Management

Radiography: Same as above

CT scan: It is helpful to detect collapse of scaphoid.

MRI: It can detect the fracture and the signs of vascularity. The proximal fragment shows low signal intensity on T_1- and T_2- weighted images of MRI of wrist.

Bone scan: It shows area of decreased uptake of radioactive material.

Treatment

- Open reduction and internal fixation with Herbert screws with bone grafting. The bone grafting can be taken from iliac crest (non-vascularized bone grafting) or locally from distal end radius with intact vascular supply (vascularized bone grafting).
- If there is associated mild arthritis: The options include:
  a. Radial styloidectomy, i.e. removal radial styloid.
  b. Proximal row carpectomy, i.e. removal of proximal row of carpal bones.
  c. Partial fusion of wrist bones.
- When there is associated advanced arthritis: Complete wrist fusion is required.

Q10. Write a short note on management of fracture scaphoid.

(10, BFUHS November 2013)

Ans: Write down first the investigations and treatment mentioned under fracture scaphoid (question number 8) and then investigations and treatment under non-union fracture scaphoid (question number 9).

Q11. Write a short note on Monteggia fracture.

(5, BFUHS May 2018, 5, BFUHS November 2011, 3, DU)

Ans: Monteggia fracture dislocation involves dislocation of head of radius with fracture of shaft of upper one-third of ulna.

Mechanism or mode of injury
• Fall on outstretched hand with forearm in pronation.
• Direct trauma

Clinical features
Symptoms
• Pain and swelling over the proximal end of forearm
• Inability to move at elbow

Signs
• Tenderness over the proximal ulna
• Radial can be palpated in abnormal position on movement.
• The distal neurovascular assessment should be thoroughly carried out as there are chances of radial nerve injury.

Diagnosis: Anteroposterior and lateral radiograph of forearm with elbow and wrist can diagnose the fracture and dislocation.

Classification: The Monteggia fracture is classified depending upon the direction of dislocation of radial head as follows:
• *Type I*: Anterior dislocation of radial head with ulnar fracture.
• *Type II*: Posterior dislocation of radial head with ulnar fracture.
• *Type III*: Lateral dislocation of radial head with ulnar fracture
• *Type IV*: Anterior dislocation of radial head with fracture of both bone forearm.

Treatment
Non-operative: In children, the closed reduction and plaster of Paris slab is applied for 6 weeks.
Operative: In adults, open reduction and internal fixation of ulnar fracture is carried out. The radial head

is relocated in majority of the cases. Few cases, however require open reduction of radial head.

Complications

1. Malunion of ulna
2. Non-union of ulna
3. Persistence dislocation of radial head
4. Stiffness around elbow joint
5. Heterotopic ossification around elbow

Q12. Write a short note on pulled elbow?

(1, RJ January 2008)

Ans: It is usually encountered in children between the ages of 2 to 5 years.

Mechanism of injury: Pulling the forearm in pronation leads to radial head dislocation.

Clinical features
Symptoms: Pain and swelling over the elbow. There is no movement possible at elbow.

Signs

• The forearm lies in attitude of pronation
• Tenderness over the lateral aspect of elbow

Diagnosis: The diagnosis is mainly clinical. X-ray of elbow may not detect the radial head dislocation due to its cartilaginous nature.

Treatment: Traction given along the forearm and simultaneously supinated, the radial head relocates usually with sound of a click.

Q13. Write a short note on cubitus varus.

(5, BFUHS November 2007, 5,
BFUHS May 2010, 5, BFUHS,
May 2011, 1, RJ, January 2011)
Or
Write a short note on gunstock deformity.

(1, RJ January 2009)

Ans: It is a deformity in which there is inward deviation of forearm.

Etiology

1. Cubitus varus is malunited supracondylar humerus (most common)
2. Avascular necrosis of trochlea.

Pathoanatomy: The deformity involves loss of coronal alignment to make the distal forearm and hand deviate to the midline of the body and recurvatum deformation in the sagittal plane and internal rotation deformity in the axial plane. Recurvatum deformity is in the plane of motion of the joint and remodels well. The internal rotation deformity is compensated by shoulder movements and is tolerated well. Both these deformities may not require corrections and most of the times correction is focused on coronal plane deformity.

Clinical features: The range of motion at the elbow joint is normal. It is only a cosmetic deformity. However, the chances of lateral condyle fracture and tardy ulnar nerve palsy.

X-ray: Anteroposterior and lateral views help in assessing the amount of deformity and surgical planning.

Treatment

- Corrective osteotomy is carried out approximately one year after injury
- *Surgical options are*
  1. Lateral closing wedge osteotomy
  2. French modified osteotomy
  3. Medial open wedge osteotomy
  4. Step cut osteotomy
  5. Dome osteotomy

Q14. Write a short note on cubitus valgus. (3, *DU*)

Ans: When forearm is angled away from the body greater than normal in a fully extended elbow, it is called cubitus valgus.

Etiology

- Osteonecrosis of lateral trochlea
- Malunited intercondylar fracture

- Radial head fracture dislocation
- Medial epiphyseal injury
- Turner syndrome
- Noonan syndrome

Clinical features
- Deformity at elbow
- Range of motion is almost equal to other limb
- Tardy ulnar nerve palsy in some cases

Investigations
X-ray: It confirms the diagnosis and helps in surgical planning.

Treatment
- Medial closing wedge osteotomy
- Dome osteotomy
- Step cut osteotomy

Q15. Write a short note on Galeazzi fracture.

(2, RJ January 2016, 3, DU)

Ans: Definition: It involves the fracture involving distal one-third of the radius shaft and distal radioulnar joint (DRUJ) disruption.

Mechanism of injury
- Direct trauma
- Indirect injury: Fall on outstretched hand

Clinical features
Symptoms
- Pain
- Swelling

Signs
- Deformity of forearm
- Point tenderness over the forearm
- Swelling of forearm
- Prominence of lower end of ulna.

   Radiograph of forearm shows fracture is seen in the lower third of the radius. The distal radioulnar joint is subluxated or dislocated which is demonstrated on X-ray as dorsal or volar displacement of ulnar head and shortening of radius by more than 5 mm.

Treatment

• Closed reduction in children.

• Open reduction and internal fixation with plating of radius restores the radial and distal radioulnar joint is addressed in following ways:

a. The distal radioulnar joint is reduced and stable: No further action is needed. The arm is rested for a few days, and then gentle active movements are encouraged. The radioulnar joint should be checked, both clinically and radiologically, during the next 6 weeks.

b. The distal radioulnar joint is reduced but unstable. The forearm should be immobilized in the position of stability (usually supination), supplemented if required by a transverse K-wire. The forearm is splinted in an above-elbow cast for 6 weeks. If there is a large ulnar styloid fragment, it should be reduced and fixed.

c. The distal radioulnar joint is irreducible. Open reduction is needed to remove the interposed soft tissues. The triangular fibrocartilage complex (TFCC) and dorsal capsule are then carefully repaired and the forearm immobilized in the position of stability (again, usually supination, supported by a wire if needed) for 6 weeks.

Q16. Write a short note on Bennett's fracture.

(2, RJ January 2012)

Ans: It is oblique intra-articular fracture of the base of the first metacarpal with subluxation or dislocation of the metacarpal.

Mechanism of injury: The axial blow directed against partially flexed metacarpal results in fracture dislocation.

Clinical features

There is pain, swelling and tenderness over the base of first metacarpal.

Treatment

Accurate reduction and restoration of the smooth joint surface is very important because this being an intra-articular fracture. If not reduced accurately, it may lead to incongruity of the articular surfaces and would increase the chance of osteoarthritis.

It is often possible to achieve reduction by manipulation under anesthesia. Following methods of treatment are used:

1. Closed manipulation and plaster cast.
2. Closed reduction and percutaneous fixation under X-ray control using an image intensifier.
3. Open reduction and internal fixation using K-wire or a screw.

Q17. Write a short note on fracture of lateral condyle of humerus. (3, DU)

Ans: This is a common fracture in children, results from a varus injury to the elbow. The fractured fragments comprise capitulum and lateral condyle. The fracture line runs obliquely upwards and laterally from the intercondylar area.

Clinical features

• There is history of fall on an outstretched hand.
• There is pain and swelling over the lateral aspect of elbow.
• The pain is increased on wrist flexion or extension.
• There is tenderness over the lateral aspect of the distal humerus.

Classification on X-ray

Type 1: Displacement of fracture of less than 2 mm, indicating intact cartilaginous hinge.

Type 2: Displacement of fracture fragment between 2 mm and 4 mm with intact articular cartilage on arthrogram.

Type 3: Displacement of fracture fragment by more than 4 mm and articular surface disrupted on arthrogram

Treatment: Appropriate reduction of fracture is important. Treatment depends upon whether the fracture is displaced or not.

A. An undisplaced fracture needs support in an elbow plaster slab for 2–3 weeks.

B. A displaced fracture is treated by open reduction and internal fracture by two K-wires and the Kirschner's wire are removed at 6 weeks.

Complications

1. Non-union
2. Delayed union
3. Cubitus valgus deformity with or without tardy nerve palsy
4. Cubitus varus
5. Avascular necrosis
6. Lateral overgrowth or prominence
7. Growth arrest.

Chapter 5

Lower Limb and Spine Injuries

Q1. Describe signs and symptoms of fracture neck of femur and its management in a 70-year-old.

(10, BFUHS November 2007)

Or

Describe in detail the management of femur fracture in 30-year-old. *(5, BFUHS November 2008)*

Or

Write a short note on treatment of fracture neck of femur in adults. *(5, BFUHS November 2017)*

Or

Describe in detail fracture neck femur and its complications and management.

(10, BFUHS May 2009)

Or

Diagnosis, management and complications of fracture neck femur. *(10, BFUHS May 2011)*

Or0

Management of fracture neck of femur in adult age group. *(2.5, RJ, 2015)*

Or

Clinical features and management of fracture neck of femur. *(3, DU)*

Ans: Majority of the fracture neck of femur occurs in elderly population and few cases of young and children are seen with this fracture.

Mechanism or mode of injury

- *In elderly:* Low energy trauma like fall in washroom, fall while walking can lead to fracture neck of femur.
- *In young adults:* High energy trauma like motor vehicular accident or fall from height.

Clinical features

Symptoms

- Pain and swelling in the hip region.
- Inability to bear weight over the leg

Signs

- Limb is shortened and externally rotated.
- Tenderness over the greater trochanter.
- In neglected cases, Trendelenburg test is positive.

Diagnosis

- Anteroposterior and lateral radiograph of hip can detect and classify the fracture.
- Undisplaced fracture can be diagnosed with help of MRI and CT scan.

Classifications: Three commonly used classifications used to classify fracture neck of femur are:

1. *Garden's classification*

   Type I: It is incomplete (fracture line does not break the medial cortex) fracture.

   Type II: Complete but undisplaced

   Type III: Complete but partially displaced

   Type IV: Complete fracture and fully displaced.

2. *Anatomical classification*

   - *Subcapital:* Fracture just below the head
   - *Transcervical:* Fracture through middle of the neck of femur
   - *Basicervical:* Fracture through base of neck of femur.

3. *Pauwel's classification:* It based upon the angle formed between fracture line and horizontal

   Type I: Less than 30° from horizontal

Type II: Angle between 30° and 50° from horizontal
Type III: Angle more than 50° from horizontal.

Management

Young adults and children

- In fresh cases (less than three months old): Closed reduction and internal fixation with cannulated cancellous screws or dynamic hip screw.
- In old neglected cases (more than 3 months old):
  - Valgus subtrochanteric osteotomy.
  - McMurray's osteotomy
  - Vascularized muscle pedicle bone grafting.

Elderly population

- In fresh cases, closed reduction and internal fixation with cannulated cancellous screws or dynamic hip screws can be chosen in individuals with age less than 65 years.
- In old neglected cases and patients with age greater than 65 years require hemi or total hip replacement.

Hemiarthroplasty or half hip replacement

- It is indicated in individuals with no signs of osteoarthritis in acetabulum.
- Austin Moore and Thompson's prosthesis are two commonly used implants for hemiarthroplasty.

Total hip replacement: In case the acetabulum shows signs of arthritis complete hip is replaced.

Complications

- Non-union: It is the most common complication encountered in fracture neck of femur.
- Avascular necrosis of head of femur. Due to disruption of blood supply at neck of femur. The femoral head can undergo avascular necrosis.
- Secondary osteoarthritis of hip joint subsequent to avascular necrosis of hip.

Q2. Write a short note on blood supply of neck of femur.

(3, *DU*)

Ans: The blood supply to femoral neck and head is mainly through the branches of the femoral artery.

a. Extracapsular arterial ring at the base of the femoral neck:

It is formed by contribution following three arterial branches:

1. Posteriorly by large branch of medial femoral circumflex artery.

2. Anteriorly by smaller branches of lateral femoral circumflex artery.

3. Superiorly and inferiorly by minor contributions by gluteal artery.

b. *Ascending cervical branches:* The arteries ascending from the extracapsular arterial ring at the base of femoral neck gives rise to retinacular arteries, namely superior, inferior, posterior and anterior.

c. *Artery of ligamentum teres:* It is mainly a branch arising from obturator artery and rarely from medial femoral circumflex artery. It forms only approximately 20% of the blood supply as majority of the blood supply is from the extracapsular arterial ring.

d. *Epiphyseal blood supply:* Some tiny lateral epiphyseal arteries enter posterosuperiorly through head of femur.

e. *Metaphyseal blood supply:* It arises from the extra-articular arterial ring and supplies the metaphyseal region.

Q3. Complications of fracture neck of femur.

(5, *BFUHS November 2009, 2, RJ January 2012, 2, RJ January 2013*)

Ans: The complications of fracture include osteonecrosis, non-union, secondary osteoarthritis and implant failure in case of treated fractures.

a. **Osteonecrosis**

• The chances of osteonecrosis or avascular necrosis are due the precarious blood supply of head of femur.

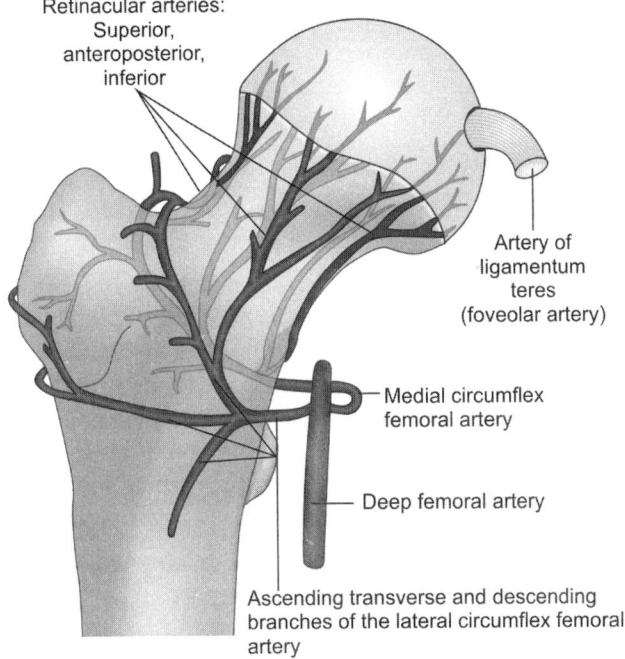

Retinacular arteries:
Superior,
anteroposterior,
inferior

Artery of
ligamentum
teres
(foveolar artery)

Medial circumflex
femoral artery

Deep femoral artery

Ascending transverse and descending
branches of the lateral circumflex femoral
artery

- The incidence is between 10 and 45%
- It can develop even in cases of undisplaced and accurate reduction and fixation of the fracture. However, the risk of avascular necrosis is higher in cases of marked initial displacement and non-anatomic reduction or malreduced fracture.
- **Treatment of osteonecrosis**
    - *In young adults*: Vascularized fibular grafting or total hip replacement in selected cases.
    - *In elderly population*: Hemiarthroplasty or total hip replacement depending upon the individual case.

b. **Non-union**
    - The chances of non-union are high in cases with high initial displacement at the time of injury.

• The incidence is between 5 and 30%.

• High incidence of non-union is seen in cases of fracture fixed initially in varus, i.e. angle between femoral neck and shaft is lower than the normal side.

Treatment

• If the vascular supply to the head of femur is maintained:

Valgus intertrochanteric osteotomy: In this procedure the lateral wedge from the proximal femur is removed and fixed with increased femoral neck shaft angle (hence called valgus) and vertical fracture line is converted into horizontal. So, the shearing vertical forces are now converted to horizontal compression forces.

• In the vascular supply to the head of femur is compromised:

1. Free vascularized fibular graft is passed across the fracture site from lateral aspect of femur into femoral head.

2. Arthroplasty: The replacement of non-viable femoral head with prosthesis is the other available option.

c. *Secondary osteoarthritis:* It may develop in case of non-viable or femoral head with no vascular supply. It may occur in treated or neglected non-treated cases of fracture femur neck non-union. The treatment of secondary osteoarthritis is total hip replacement.

d. *Implant failure:* In some cases, the initial fixation of the fracture with cannulated cancellous screws or other implants may fail. In those cases depending upon the viability of femoral head the treatment modality is chosen (as mentioned under femoral neck non-union above).

Q4. Write a short note on complication of fracture shaft of femur. *(5, BFUHS May 2018)*

Ans: Complications of fracture shaft of femur include:

1. *Malunion:* It may be encountered in cases managed non-operatively and operatively. Rotational malalignment can occur especially in comminuted fractures due to lack of recognizable bony landmarks. During operative procedure the limb alignment can be assessed intraoperative fluoroscopy. Rotational malalignment of greater than 20° require operative correction. Mild sagittal malalignment is tolerable while coronal malalignment is not as it can severely compromise limb function.

2. *Non-union:* Femur is surrounded by strong bellies of the thigh muscles. The muscular pull leads to the formation of gap between the bony ends. In case of surgical treatment, improper handling of soft tissues and suboptimal implant selection can lead to femoral union.

3. *Fat emboli syndrome:* Femoral shaft fracture can result in fat embolism in rare cases. It is a medical emergency to manage.

   Pathophysiology: It usually presents after 48 hours after the injury. There is migration of fat globules from the fracture site into the blood circulation. The fat globule migration can be encountered during reaming in femoral nailing.

   Clinical presentation: It presents as respiratory distress, petechiae over the skin, drowsiness. There is significant associated morbidity and mortality.

   Treatment: High flow oxygenation and low molecular weight heparin are used to treat the condition.

4. *Deep vein thrombosis:* Due to prolonged immobilization especially in conservatively managed cases, there are chances of deep vein thrombosis and subsequent pulmonary embolization.

5. *Sciatic neurapraxia:* Rarely it is seen in cases of femoral shaft fracture. It is usually seen in case of retrograde nailing with proximal migration of pin or nail.

6. *Infection:* In some cases treated operatively, there are chances of infection of bone presenting as osteomyelitis.

7. *Quadriceps contracture:* It is seen in conservatively managed cases or in cases where mobilization at knee is delayed after operative fixation. It can be prevented with mobilization at the knee joint right after the surgical management.

Q5. Discuss mechanism of injury of patella and discuss its management. (5, *Rajasthan January 2016*)

Or

Write a short note on fracture patella. (3, *DU*)

Ans: The patella is a sesamoid bone in continuity with the quadriceps tendon and the patellar ligament. The mechanical function of the patella is to hold the entire extensor 'strap' away from the center of rotation of the knee, thereby lengthening the anterior lever arm and increasing the efficiency of the quadriceps.

Mechanism of injury: The patella may be fractured, either by a direct force that cracks the bone like a tile under the blow of a hammer or by an indirect traction force that pulls the bone apart.

- Direct injury—usually a fall onto the knee or a blow against the dashboard of a car—causes either an undisplaced crack or else a comminuted ('stellate') fracture without severe damage to the extensor expansions.

- Indirect injury occurs, typically, when someone catches the foot against a solid obstacle and, to avoid falling, contracts the quadriceps muscle forcefully. This causes a transverse fracture with a gap between the fragments.

Clinical features
- The knee becomes swollen and painful.
- The patella is tender and sometimes a gap can be felt.
- Active knee extension should be tested. If the patient can lift the straight leg, the quadriceps mechanism is still intact. If this maneuver is too painful, active extension can be tested with the patient lying on his/her side.

Classification
It can be classified as:
- Nondisplaced
- Transverse
- Vertical
- Comminuted

Radiographic diagnosis: The X-ray may show one or more fine fracture lines without displacement, multiple fracture lines with irregular displacement or a transverse fracture with a gap between the fragments.

Treatment
- *Non-operative:* Knee is immobilized with the help of brace or cylinder cast.

  Indications for non-operative management:
  - Intact extensor mechanism which can be diagnosed by asking the patient to do straight leg raise
  - Nondisplaced or minimally displaced fractures
  - Vertical fracture patterns
- *Operative*
  a. *Open reduction and internal fixation*
     - Indications
       - Extensor mechanism failure (unable to perform straight leg raise)
       - Open fractures

- Fracture articular displacement >2 mm
- Displaced patella fracture >3 mm
  - Methods of internal reduction and internal fixation:
    - Tension band with Kirschner wire and cerclage wire.
    - Minifragment with lag screws
  b. *Partial patellectomy*
    - Indications
      - Comminuted patella fracture with one big chunk intact either superior or inferior pole.
  c. *Total patellectomy*
    - Indication:
      - Comminuted patella fracture which cannot be reconstructed.

Q6. Write a short note on diagnosis, clinical signs and complications of posterior dislocation of hip.

(3, DU)

Ans: Hip joint is inherently stable due to labrum, capsule and ligaments like iliofemoral ligament.

- **Mechanism of injury:** When someone seated in a truck or car is thrown forward, striking the knee against the dashboard. The femur is thrust upwards and the femoral head is forced out of its socket.
- **Clinical features**
  - *Symptoms:* Pain and inability to bear weight.
  - *Signs:* Hip and leg are in flexion, adduction, and internal rotation.
- **Associated injuries:** There may be associated injuries with posterior hip dislocation:
  - Posterior wall or column fracture of acetabulum.
  - Fracture of neck or head of femur.
  - Knee ligament injuries
  - Neurovascular injury (sciatic nerve injury is most commonly affected)
  - Chest injuries as it is usually high impact injury.

- **Diagnosis**
  - *Radiograph*: In the anteroposterior film the femoral head is seen out of its socket and above the acetabulum. A segment of acetabular rim or femoral head may have been broken off and displaced. CT scan is the best way of demonstrating an associated acetabular fracture.
- **Treatment**
  - *Non-operative treatment:* Patient is given sedation and muscle relaxant to aid in reduction. The dislocation must be reduced as soon as possible generally within six hours to reduce the risk of avascular necrosis of femoral head. An assistant steadies the pelvis; the surgeon starts by applying traction in the line of the femur as it lies (usually in adduction and internal rotation), and then gradually flexes the patient's hip and knee to 90 °, maintaining traction throughout. At 90° of hip flexion, traction is steadily increased and sometimes a little rotation (either internal or external) is required to accomplish reduction. Movement and exercises were begun as soon as pain allows.
  - *Operative treatment:* In some cases when closed reduction is not possible due to inverted labrum or intra-articular fragment, the hip is approached anteriorly through Smith Peterson approach.
- **Complications**
  - *Early*:
    - Sciatic nerve injury
    - Vascular injury
  - *Late*:
    - Avascular necrosis
    - Myositis ossificans
    - Unreduced dislocation
    - Osteoarthritis

Chapter 6

Bone and Joint Infection

Q1. Write a short note on acute osteomyelitis.

(3, DU, 3, DU)

Or

Write a short note on pathogenesis of acute osteo-myelitis. (5, BFUHS May 2018)

Or

Management of acute osteomyelitis. (3, DU, 3, DU)

Or

Enumerate the complications of acute pyogenic osteomyelitis. (3, DU)

Or

Discuss the management of acute osteomyelitis of upper end of tibia in a child. (10, BFUHS May 2013)

Or

Describe pathophysiology, clinical features and treatment of acute hematogenous osteomyelitis in children. (5, RJ January 2013)

Or

Pathophysiology of pyogenic osteomyelitis. (3, DU)

Or

Discuss treatment of acute osteomyelitis. (3, DU)

Or

Pathophysiology of pyogenic osteomyelitis. (3, DU)

Or

Discuss treatment of acute osteomyelitis. (3, DU)

Ans: Definition: Bone infection presenting early mostly within two weeks of onset known as acute osteomyelitis.

Etiopathogenesis: Metaphysis of long bones is very vascularized area. Vessels in this area of bone are arranged in form of loop (hair pin arrangements). This arrangement leads to blood stasis in this area and bacteria settle there easily. Organism reaches bone mostly by blood circulation.

Commonest organism: *Staphylococcus aureus.*

Common sites of infection: Lower end of femur, upper tibia, upper femur, upper humeral end.

Pathology: Bone starts inflammatory reaction in response to bacteria in bone. This leads to bone destruction and production of pus. Whenever there is sufficient pus formation in medullary cavity it can spread in various directions:

• Along medullary cavity.

• *Out of bone cortex*: Pus travel along Volkmann's canal and lift off periosteum from underlying bone. This pus under periosteum generates new bone this phenomenon is known as periosteal reaction.

• *Other directions*: Epiphyseal plate prevents pus from entering joint. But joints with intra-articular metaphysis as in hip and shoulder joints, pus can spread to joints.

Symptoms

• Child presents with acute onset of pain and swelling at the site of infection.

• Child is reluctant to wear weight in lower limb infection case.

• Systemic feature of infection as fever.

Signs

• Redness and tenderness at the site of infection.

• Increased temperature at the site of infection.

• Systemic feature of infection as dehydration, lethargic, etc.

- If child presents late, there may be abscess formation in muscle and subcutaneous plane.
- Swelling of adjacent joint because of spread of pus/sympathetic effusion of joint.

Diagnosis

- Diagnosis of acute osteomyelitis is mainly clinical.
- *Blood investigations:* Increased TLC with rise of polymorphs. Increased ESR and CRP decreased Hb.
- *Blood culture and gram stain:* May yield causative organism.
- *X-ray:* Periosteum reaction (may take 7–10 days to appear)
- *MRI:* Rarely carried out. Medullary edema can be appreciated within 48 hours.
- Aspiration of pus from bone using thick needle.

Treatment: Child should be treated as emergency case, should be admitted immediately and routine investigation should be sent along with blood culture before starting antibiotics. Treatment also depends upon after how long of illness patient is bought to hospital, it can be divided into two main categories.

Within 48 hours of onset of symptoms: If patient is bought within 48 hours of onset of symptoms it generally means pus has not formed till now and conservative treatment is all required, patient should be admitted on emergency basis.

1. Start intravenous fluids Ringer lactate/normal saline/dextrose normal saline to rehydrate the child.
2. Splintage of affected bone with cramer wire splint/POP splint/skin traction.
3. Regular temperature/pulse recording.
4. Intravenous (IV) antibiotics only after blood culture sample as sending blood culture after starting IV antibiotics may yield negative report. Empirical antibiotics may be started as:
   a. *Child less than 4-month-old:* Ceftriaxone + vanco-mycin + amikacin

  b. *Older child*: Ceftriaxone + cloxacillin + amikacin
  c. Intravenous antibiotics should be changed according to blood culture report subsequently.
  d. Intravenous antibiotics can be changed to oral formulations after two weeks.
5. If patient does not respond to IV antibiotics within 2 days (decreased temperature decreased CBC, CRP) surgical intervention may be required
6. All cases should be serially monitored with CRP, blood counts (total leukocyte count and differential leukocyte count) everyday and ESR every weekly.
7. Pain killer to decrease pain and inflammation.

Patient presenting after 48 hours of onset of symptoms
If patient presents late or if he/she does not respond to IV antibiotics, it generally means that pus has already formed in or outside bone, and it may require surgical exploration and pus removal from bone after making multiple drill holes in bone, sterile suction drain is applied before closure. Splintage, IV antibiotics and IV fluids should be given.

Complications
These can be general and local complications.

General complications: Patient may develop pyrexia and septicemia, dehydration, if patient is malnourished these can prove fatal, patient can go to septicemic shock and organ failure.

Local complications: These are those which limit to local body part that is effected by acute osteomyelitis, these can be:

  a. *Chronic osteomyelitis* is most common complication of acute osteomyelitis. Delay in treatment especially in malnourished child leads to more pus formation in medullary cavity which can come out of bone and skin after forming sinus.
  b. *Acute pyogenic arthritis*: Pus can travel to nearby joint especially where metaphysic is intra-articular, e.g. hip and shoulder joints, leading to pyogenic arthritis, which can damage joint and cause joint stiffness.

c. *Growth disturbances*: Pus can damage epiphysis partially or completely which can lead to growth disturbances.

d. *Pathological fractures*: Pus can lead to bone weakness so patient can have fracture of that part of bone after minor trauma.

Q2. Describe the etiopathogenesis, clinical features, complications and treatment of chronic osteomyelitis.

(10, BFUHS May 2010)

Or

Describe pathological and radiological features of chronic osteomyelitis and also discuss complications of chronic osteomyelitis. *(10, BFUHS May 2014)*

Or

Chronic osteomyelitis. *(7, BFUHS May 2008)*

Or

Define osteomyelitis. Discuss clinical features and management of chronic osteomyelitis.

(10, RJ January 2011)

Or

Chronic osteomyelitis *(2.5, RJ December 2013)*

Or

Describe clinical features and treatment of chronic osteomyelitis in adults. *(5, RJ January 2015)*

Or

Management of chronic osteomyelitis. *(3, DU)*

Or

Complications of chronic osteomyelitis.

(5, RJ January 2012)

Or

Complications of chronic osteomyelitis.

(5, BFUHS November 2007)

Or

Discuss the complications of chronic osteomyelitis and their management. *(10, BFUHS May 2016)*

Or

Write a short note on treatment principles of chronic osteomyelitis, both surgical and medical and also discuss about complications of chronic osteomyelitis.

(5, BFUHS May 2017)

Ans: Bone infection caused by microorganism that present late mainly with discharging sinus is known as chronic osteomyelitis.

Etiopathogenesis: Chronic osteomyelitis can present as:

1. Chronic osteomyelitis results most commonly as a complication of acute osteomyelitis.

2. Brodie's abscess

3. Garre's osteomyelitis

Various reasons that lead acute osteomyelitis to chronic osteomyelitis:

1. Late and inadequate treatment is the most common cause. In developing countries like India, child presents to hospital in late stage and does not take proper treatment which cause persistence of microorganism in bone and there is regular pus formation which goes on to spread in multiple directions. This leads to the formation of dead bone (sequestrum) surrounded with pus formation.

2. Decreased host resistance: Malnutrition and associated chronic illness as diabetes/rheumatoid arthritis/patient on steroid or chemotherapy/HIV which decreases immune response of body and persistence of organism in bone leading to chronic osteomyelitis. In conditions like diabetes, bone does not get a steady blood supply, so antibiotics do not reach in proper dose at site of infection.

3. In conditions such as compound fracture/fracture fixation with implant/joint replacement, there can be chances of infection if sterility of operation theatre is not maintained or host resistance is compromised. The infection can lead to chronic osteomyelitis. Host bone responds by forming more and more subperiosteal new bone leading to bone thickening, new subperiosteal bone is deposited in very irregular

fashion leading to irregular surface in chronic osteomyelitis. Continuous discharge of pus leads to sinus formation. Subsequently, sinus get fibrosed and fixed to bone with time.

Clinical features

Signs

1. Patient presents with discharging sinus from which continuously discharge is coming out. It may heal in between and reappear again after a few days.
2. *Pain*: It may or may not be present. Pain is generally associated with acute exacerbations.
3. Patient may present with generalized signs of infection like fever, malaise, weight loss, etc.

Symptoms

1. Chronic discharging sinus: It is the most important symptom presents in chronic osteomyelitis. Granulation tissue or dead pieces of bone may be coming out of it.
2. Tenderness on palpation
3. Swelling of limb with thickened irregular bone.
4. Stiffness of adjacent joint.

Management

Investigations

- *X-rays:* Irregular and thickened cortex of bone.
  - Honeycombed appearance
  - Sequestrum/involucrum/cloacae may appear
- *Blood:* ESR and TLC may be raised or within normal limit.
- Pus culture may be negative as patient may be already on antibiotics. Pus culture should be sent before starting antibiotics.
- *MRI/CT:* These are very useful to know the extent of involvement of bone and planning surgery for the chronic osteomyelitis.

Treatment

Goal: To achieve viable and bleeding bone margins which are free from infection by removing all dead bone and soft tissue and sinus tract. It can be achieved by following ways:

1. *Sequestrectomy:* It means removal of dead (sequestrum) bone. Multiple drill holes are done and part of dead bone is removed. If there is much of bone removed which can fracture bone, external fixator/ ilizarov should be applied to aid stability.

2. *Saucerization:* While removing a saucer-shaped cavity is created so that all dead bone and pus can be evacuated. Dead bone is removed till the bleeding margins of bone start appearing. Bleeding ends mean healthy bone.

3. Curettage and excision of sinus tract; all dead and infected soft tissue is removed along with sinus tract.

4. *Amputation:* It is rarely done for long bones. Amputation of toes can be done in chronic osteomyelitis in diabetic foot infections.

Complications

1. *Flare up of infection may occur:* Flare up of infection can occur commonly. It subsides with antibiotics and rest.

2. *Pathological fracture:* As bone get weakened by chronic osteomyelitis. Minor trauma/fall can cause fracture in infected bone.

3. *Adjacent joint stiffness/septic arthritis:* Infection from bone can spread to joint and there may occur scarring of soft tissue around bone and joint leading to joint stiffness. Joint destruction after septic arthritis can also cause joint stiffness and painful movement at joint.

4. Growth abnormalities in case of child with infection near epiphysis; it can present as:

a. *Shortening:* If growth plate is damaged by infection
b. *Lengthening:* Due to hyperemia (increased blood supply) to growth plate.
c. *Deformity:* If half of growth plate is damaged or half having increased blood supply and other half is not affected. So, it causes half of epiphysis to either grow more or grow less as compared to other half which is growing normal.

5. *Sinus tract malignancy:* Rare complication. It takes many years to develop after onset of osteomyelitis and if not treated. It is usually squamous cell carcinoma.

6. Amyloidosis: It is late complication of osteomyelitis.

Q3. Write a short note on sequestrum

(5, BFUHS May 2011)

Ans: Sequestrum is a piece of dead bone that has become separated during the process of necrosis from normal or sound bone. It is a complication of osteomyelitis.

Pathology: Infection in bone leads to increase in intra-medullary pressure due to collection of inflammatory exudates in response to infection. Periosteum is striped from osteum, leading to vascular thrombosis. This leads to lack of blood supply and bone necrosis which further leads to sequestrum formation. Sequestrum has smooth inner and rough outer surface because outer surface is constantly eroded by the surrounding granulation tissue. Dense sclerotic bone overlying sequestrum is known as involucrum. There may be holes in involucrum to drain out pus these are known as cloacae.

Different types of sequestra
- *Tuberculosis:* Feathery, flake, coarse sandy, kissing sequestra (TB knee and spine)
- *Syphilis:* Ivory
- Amputation stump/pin tract infection; ring sequestra
- *Pyogenic osteomyelitis:* Tubular or diaphyseal sequestra.

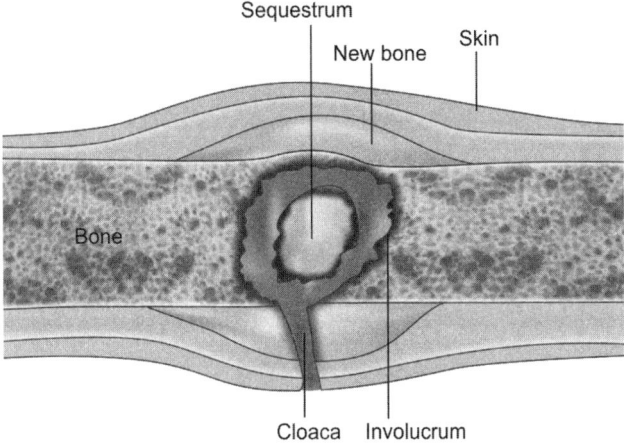

Sequestrum
New bone
Skin
Bone
Cloaca   Involucrum

- After radiation: Button hole sequestra
- Actinomycosis: Black sequestra

Management

Investigation

- *X-ray* shows dense area in bone as compared to surrounding bone. Because decalcification which occurs in normal bone, does not occur in sequestrum.
- *MRI/CT*: These are useful to know the extent of bone involvement and planning for surgery.

Treatment

Sequestrectomy: After planning for surgery on MRI. Multiple drill holes are done in bone and dead piece of bone is removed. All dead bone is removed; it is decided while operation to remove bone till there appear bleeding ends of bone. If much of bone get removed and there are chances of fracture, external fixator is applied.

Q4. Write a short note on septic arthritis knee.

(5, BFUHS November 2009, 5, BFUHS November 2008)

Or

Describe clinicoradiological signs of septic arthritis of hip and its management. *(10, BFUHS May 2007)*

Ans: Definition: Septic arthritis is a pyogenic infection of the joint, typically it is acute joint infection, but can be subacute or chronic.

Etiopathogenesis

- More common in children, mainly boys.
- Most common joint involved is knee joint.
- Predisposing conditions: Poor hygiene, malnutrition, poor resistance (diabetes, rheumatoid arthritis/ chronic disease)
- Most common organism: *Staphylococcus aureus.*

Route of transmission

1. *Hematogenous:* Commonest route
2. Secondary to nearby bone or soft tissue infection
3. Penetrating wounds
4. Iatrogenic as during intra-articular injections.

Diagnosis: It is mainly clinical.

Signs

1. Extensive pain of joint, leading to immobility of joint, patient does not allow anybody to touch the joint
2. Swelling of joint
3. Redness of joint
4. High grade fever and malaise.

Symptoms

1. Joint seems swollen.
2. On palpation; tenderness of joint, increased local temperature.
3. In knee; patellar tap test will be positive.
4. Tachycardia and high temperature.
5. Patient will keep limb in position of ease, i.e. knee in flexion with hip in flexion, abduction and external rotation.

Management

Investigations

1. *X-rays:*
   - Early stage—increased joint space due to joint effusion.

- Late stage—joint space narrowing due to destruction of articular cartilage, loss of continuity of white cortical lines as bone destruction begins and development of margin erosions as bone is further destroyed.
2. *MRI/CT/ultrasonography:* Early diagnosis of synovial thickening, soft tissue swelling.
3. Blood: Increased ESR, CRP, TLC, neutrophilia.
4. Joint fluid analysis:
   - Yellowish green color due to elevated levels of nucleated cells.
   - Microscopic examination shows increased cell counts with predominance of polymorphonuclear leukocytes.
   - Gram staining may identify the organism leading to knee arthritis.
   - Biochemical analysis shows decreased glucose levels and increased protein concentration.

Treatment

In early stage: Before joint destruction begins, treat patient as emergency.

1. Start IV fluids, IV antibiotics as cefotaxime (100–150 mg/kg/day) and amikacin (15 mg/kg/day) in divided doses. Change to antibiotics according to culture sensitivity and continue antibiotics for 6 weeks.

2. Splintage of joint.

3. If pus is coming from sinus or aspirated, arthrotomy should be done and joint should be washed and debridement by removing inflamed synovium and all pus should be done.

In late stage: If patient presents late, there will be joint destruction along with subluxation/dislocation of joint. In such cases, joint movement may not be possible or very painful. Patient may need arthrodesis of joint as in ankle/subtalar, or joint replacement as in knee and hip joint, only after complete eradication of infection.

Q5. Write a short note on Tom Smith arthritis. (3, *DU*)

Ans: It is a septic arthritis of hip during infancy, and usually follows infected umbilical cord.

Source of infection: It is mainly bloodborne. Primary source of infection is from skin, upper respiratory tract, umbilicus in newborn, paranasal sinus.

Most common microorganism: *Staphylococcus aureus*
Involvement of joint: It most commonly involves hip joint. Other knee and shoulder can also be involved. Rarely multiple joints involvement.

Presentation
- The head and neck of femur undergoes rapid destruction with resulting pathological dislocation of hip joint resulting in shortening of limb.
- On examination:
  – Shortening of lower limb.
  – Child walks with unstable gait. There is limp without pain.
  – Hip movements are restricted.
  – Telescopy test is positive.

Investigations
- *X-ray:* It may show complete absence of head and neck of femur although it may be much informative because of the cartilaginous nature of the head of femur.
- *Ultrasonography/MRI:* It can better evaluate the shape of head and neck of femur.

Treatment
- *Early presentation:* IV broad-spectrum antibiotics, traction/splintage/hip joint lavage arthroscopy/open
- *Late presentation:* Osteotomy for stabilizing hip joint.

Chapter 7

Tuberculosis

Q1. Describe etiopatholgy, presentation, investigations and management of Koch's spine at thoracolumbar junction in adults. *(5, RJ January 2013)*

Or

Discuss etiopathogenesis, management and complications of tuberculosis spine.

(5, BFUHS November 2011)

Or

Potts's paraplegia. *(4, RJ, January 2012, 3, DU)*

Or

Enumerate the clinical signs and symptoms of tuberculosis of dorsal spine. *(3, DU)*

Ans: Spinal tuberculosis or Pott's disease is one of the oldest demonstrated diseases of humankind. It is documented in spinal remains from the iron age in Europe and in ancient mummies from Egypt.

Etiopathology

- *Vertebrae affected:* Thoracolumbar junction (D10 to L2) > lumbar > cervical.

- *Source of infection to spine:* Lungs, gastrointestinal tract and genitourinary system. Mycobacteria spread to the spinal vertebrae through hematogenous route (blood).

- The bacteria lodge in the vertebra and destroy it secondary to chronic inflammation. The intervertebral disc which gets its nutrition from the vertebral body, hence is destroyed. There is wedging of the vertebrae due to its destruction which presents as kyphosis (forward bending of spine). The spinal canal can be narrowed by abscesses, granulation tissue, or direct dural invasion, leading to spinal cord compression and neurologic deficits.
- There is formation of pus in the diseases vertebrae which tracks into area of least resistance and present as cold abscess (in contrast to normal abscess which is warm and tender).

Presentation or clinical features

- *Pain:* It is commonest presenting symptom. It may be localized to the area or diffuse in nature.
- *Muscle spasm or stiffness:* The patient presents with stiffness in back due to muscle spasm which prevents the movement at spinal column.
- *Spinal deformity:* The destruction of the vertebrae leads to kyphosis (forward bending) or scoliosis (side bending).
- *Cold abscess:* The pus formed around diseased vetrebrae travels through sheath of vessels, nervous and muscular planes and can present over cervical region, chest wall, iliac fossa and popliteal fossa.
- *Neurological features:* Sometimes the pus or deformity of the involved vertebrae might present with features secondary to the pressure over the spinal cord or nerve roots. The patient might experience weakness in limbs (paraparesis) or complete loss of power (paraplegia). There could be radiating pain down the limb due to nerve root involvement.
- *Constitutional symptoms:* Like fever, malaise, weight loss and evening rise of temperature might be present in some cases.

Investigations

- *Blood:* Elevated ESR and CRP. Increased lymphocytes in TLC.
- Skin hypersensitivity testing or Mantoux test: Positive in 84–95% of patients.
- The pus obtained from the involved is subjected to AFB staining and culture. It is positive in only 50% cases.
- *CBNAAT or gene-Xpert:* It is a gene-based testing for *Mycobacterium tuberculosis* and is positive in 95% cases.
- **Radiography (X-ray findings)**
  - Decreased intervertebral disc space
  - Lytic destruction of a vertebral body
  - Wedging or collapse of vertebrae
  - Osteoporosis of the involved vertebra
  - Widening of psoas shadows (when there is involvement of lumbar vertebrae)
  - It may present as sclerosis of the involved vertebrae in healing phase.
- *Computed tomography:* Detects destruction of vertebrae in early stage of the disease.
- **Magnetic resonance imaging**
  - It detects the vertebral destruction, extent of abscess and encroachment of spinal canal with pus and vertebral deformity.
- *Biopsy:* The diseased portion of the vertebrae shows signs of chronic inflammation with granuloma formation.

Treatment

Non-operative management: The patients are advised bedrest, antitubercular therapy (ATT) and spinal braces.

- *Bedrest:* The patients are advised bedrest till the intensive phase of ATT is over. Subsequent to it the patients are allowed mobilization with spinal braces depending upon the level of vertebral involvement.

- *Antitubercular therapy*: The treatment regimen in osteoarticular tuberculosis is different from pulmonary tuberculosis. The patients are given ATT for 18 months.

  Intensive phase (3 months): It targets the extracellular fast growing bacteria. Four drugs—isoniazid (INH), rifampicin (R), pyrazinamide (Z), ethambutol (E) are given for three months.

  Continuation phase (9 months): In this phase the slow growing intracellular bacteria are targeted. Isoniazid, rifampicin and ethambutol are given.

  Prophylactic phase (6 months): In this phase the dormant bacteria are tackled. The drugs given in this phase are isoniazid and ethambutol.
- Operative treatment.

Indications

- Neurologic deficit: Progressively increasing weakness in limb.
- Bladder or bowel involvement
- No response to medical therapy.

Surgical procedure: Spinal canal decompression with removal of diseases vertebrae and drainage of abscess. The spinal canal is decompressed, i.e. removal of the diseased part of the vertebrae which is pressing upon the spinal cord or spinal root. Sometimes the vertebrae are stabilized with screws and cages after decompression to control the movement of spine.

Complications

- *Deformity*: There could be formation of kyphosis or gibbus.
- If there is involvement of cervical spine, the patient may present with retropharyngeal abscess affecting swallowing or hoarseness.
- Sinus formation
- *Paraplegia*: The patients with untreated case may lead to paraplegia.

Q2. Write a short note on cold abscess.

(5, BFUHS May 2006,
5, BFUHS May 2011, 5, BFUHS May 2003)

Ans: Definition: Cold abscess refers to an abscess that lacks the intense inflammation usually associated with infection, i.e. warmth, tenderness and fever.

Etiopathogenesis

- Cold abscess usually forms slowly over time. It forms gradually over time so there is less of pain and inflammation. Pus travels along the vessels, nerves and muscular planes and can present anywhere in the body.
- *Causative agents:* Bacteria like tuberculosis, fungi like blastomycosis, in persons suffering from hyper-immunoglobulin E syndrome Staphylococcus might cause it.

Clinical features

- *Common sites affected:* Lungs, spine, groin, pelvis and lymph nodes.
- The cold abscess especially in tuberculosis can be palpated at sides of the neck, chest wall, iliac fossa, femoral triangle and popliteal fossa.
- There is swelling with no warmth, minimal or no tenderness.

Investigations

Blood: Raised ESR and CRP

Radiograph/X-ray findings: It may present as paravertebral or prevertebral shadows depending upon the involved vertebrae.

Ultrasound: Helps in detecting the extent of the abscess.

MRI: It defines the extent of abscess and also differentiates from tumoral masses.

Aspiration cytology: It helps in identifying the organism and initiates the best treatment.

Treatment

• *Aspiration and drainage under guidance of ultrasound:* The cold abscess is drained under the guidance of ultrasound and pigtail catheter is inserted for continuous drainage.

• *Removal of the source:* As cold abscess may present in body at a site different from the site of origin. It is important to remove the diseased area and treat the organism with appropriate antibiotics.

Q3. Write a short note on compound palmar ganglion.

(3, DU)

Ans: It is tuberculous tenosynovitis of flexor tendons of wrist and hand.

Incidence

• Upper limb is more commonly involved than lower limb.

• Flexor tendons are involved usually.

Pathogenesis

• The source of infection could be direct inoculation or hematogenous spread from lungs, genitourinary tract or lymph nodes.

• It passes through three stages:

a. Formation of vascular granulation tissue.

b. Fibrosis of tendon sheath and rice bodies formation.

c. Caseation and granulation tissue formation with rupture of tendon sheath.

Clinical features

• There is swelling over the volar aspect of forearm.

• Sometimes there are symptoms of median nerve compression in advanced stages.

Differential diagnosis

• Rheumatoid arthritis

• Gouty arthritis

• Pyogenic infection

• Infected ganglion

- Sarcoidosis
- Foreign body tenosynovitis
- Fungal infection
- Pigmented villonodular synovitis of tendon sheath
- Amyloidosis

Diagnosis

- ESR is raised
- Positive Mantoux test
- MRI shows thickening of synovial sheath of tendons and fluid accumulation.
- Biopsy: Caseous necrosis, epithelial granuloma and Langhan's type giant cells.

Treatment

- Excision of infected tissue
- Tenosynovectomy
- Antitubercular therapy for six months.

Q4. Discuss etiopathogenesis of tuberculosis of hip joint in children and its management.

(10, November BFUHS 2012, 5, May BFUHS 2012)

Or

Write a short note on tubercular management of hip.

(5, BFUHS May 2018)

Ans: Tuberculosis remains a major cause of skeletal infection in developing countries. Following spine, the most common site of involvement is hip joint.

Etiopathogenesis

- The disease spreads through blood and the bacteria lodges in the hip joint most commonly in the acetabular roof followed by epiphysis and metaphyseal area.
- The disease progresses through the following stages:
    a. Stage of tubercular synovitis:
        – There is joint effusion and the affected limb is held in the position of maximum capacity, i.e. flexion, abduction and external rotation.

  – *X-ray:* There is widening of hip joint space with generalized osteopenia.
 b. Stage of early arthritis:
  – There is spasm of adductor and flexor muscles of the thigh leading to adduction and internal rotation deformity of hip with apparent shortening of the limb.
  – The shortening of the limb is less than one centimeter.
  – X-ray: Decrease in joint space and osteopenia.
 c. Stage of late arthritis:
  – There is destruction of the joint with flexion, adduction and internal rotation of the limb
  – The movement at the hip joint is markedly decreased.
  – The limb is shortened by more than one centimeter.
  – *X-ray:* Complete loss of joint space with acetabular and femoral head destruction.
 d. Stage of late arthritis with subluxation/dislocation:
  – There is adduction deformity at hip joint with flexion and internal rotation at the involved limb.
  – X-ray:
   i. *Wandering acetabulum*: The destructed femoral head may be displaced from its normal position and forms a false acetabulum higher up in iliac bone.
   ii. *Mortar and pestle*: Due to gross destruction of the acetabulum, the size of the acetabulum may be enlarged along with small femoral head remnant giving the appearance of mortar and pestle.
 c. It may present as hip dislocation.

Clinical features
• Pain in hip, deformity according to stage of disease and shortening of limb.

- Constitutional symptoms like fever, weight loss and loss of appetite.
- Cold abscess can be palpated in the groin, over the thigh and other areas.
- Muscle wasting of thigh and hip muscles.
- Anterior joint line tenderness
- Exaggerated lumbar lordosis

Differential diagnosis

- Developmental dysplasia of hip
- Congenital coxa vara
- Perthes' disease
- Septic arthritis
- Monoarticular rheumatoid arthritis

Treatment

Conservative treatment

- All patients are started on antitubercular therapy
- The affected hip is put to traction and patient is advised strict bedrest.

Operative treatment

- In case of no response to conservative treatment, the debridement of joint is carried out and the necrotic disease, inflamed synovium is removed.
- *Girdle stone arthroplasty:* The femoral head and neck is removed. It provides a painless mobile but unstable hip. However, it leads to instability and shortening.
- *Arthrodesis:* In case of painful hip, the arthrodesis is offered in some cases.

Chapter 8

Bone Tumors

Q1. Write a short note on treatment of Ewing's tumor.
(5, BFUHS November 2017)

Or

Write a short note on Ewing's sarcoma.
(5, BFUHS May 2006, BFUHS, May 2007, BFUHS November 2008, BFUHS November 2011, BFUHS May 2014, 3, DU, 3, DU)

Or

Describe clinical features and investigations in Ewing's sarcoma. *(5, RJ January 2015)*

Or

Describe the signs, symptoms and radiological appearance of Ewing's sarcoma. *(3, DU)*

Ans: Ewing's sarcoma is a malignant small cell round cell tumor.

Etiology: Various chromosomal translocations are postulated as causative agent but translocation between chromosome number 11 and 22 results in formation of EWS gene which is the oncogene.

Age group
• Most common malignant tumor under the age of 10 years.

- Second most common tumor after osteosarcoma in young adults.

Site of involvement

- Diaphysis (sometimes extending into metaphyseal region) of long bones (femur, humerus).
- Flat bones like pelvis

Clinical features

- Chief complaint is the pain. The pain is severe in nature and worse at night.
- Some patients complain of fever.
- Examination: Overlying skin is red, warm and tender. The affected site is swollen. The clinical features often are like those of acute osteomyelitis.

Investigations

Blood: Anemia, elevated ESR, leukocytosis.

Radiological

- Lytic lesion presents in the diaphyseal region of the bones with destruction of cortex and periosteal reaction (new bone formation) known as onion peel appearance.
- The lytic lesion is permeative, i.e. the lesion has small multiple defects appearing on radiographs known as moth eaten appearance.
- There is often soft tissue mass visible near to the affected area.
- Sometimes sclerotic lesions may be seen instead of lytic lesions.
- In few cases it may show features like Codman's triangle which is due to elevation of periosteum at the margins of the lesion and sunburst appearance (both these features are also seen in osteosarcoma).

Computed tomography findings: To asses cortical destruction, extent and metastasis of tumor.

Magnetic resonance imaging: Better than CT and X-ray as it.

- Provides information regarding the intramedullary extension of the tumor and soft tissue involvement.
- Helps in surgical planning before excision of the tumor.

Pathology

Gross

- Firm, greyish white with encapsulation.
- Highly vascular tumor with hemorrhage and necrosis.
- Visible cortical destruction.

Microscopy

- Small blue round cells with minimal intercellular matrix form rosettes (cells surround a central lumen to appear as floral design).
- Cells have small amount cytoplasm which is rich in glycogen and round nuclei.

Immunocytochemistry

- Like all small blue cell tumors (or primitive neuroectodermal tumors) it is positive for S-100 and neuron-specific enolase.
- It is CD99 positive, PAS positive (due to glycogen in cytoplasm) and reticulin negative.

Differential diagnosis: Chronic osteomyelitis (in chronic osteomyelitis there is sequestrum formation, mainly located in metaphysis and cloacae formation).

Treatment

The treatment of choice is first chemotherapy (vincristine, adriamycin and cyclophosphamide) for 3 to 4 weeks followed by radical resection of the tumor and then again chemotherapy along with radiotherapy.

The tumor is highly radiosensitive and it is said to "melt like snow" when radiotherapy is given but recurs again so it is not used exclusively in the primary management.

Prognosis: Bad as there are high chances of distant skeletal metastasis and generally advanced at presentation.

Bad prognostic factors

- Fever, anemia and elevated ESR, WBC count and lactate dehydrogenase.
- Distant metastasis
- Old age at presentation
- Male gender
- Involvement of pelvic bone.

Q2. Write a short note on giant cell tumor.

(5, BFUHS May 2009, BFUHS November 2010, 2, RJ January 2016, 5 RJ January 2012, 3, DU)

Or

Write a short note on treatment of giant cell tumor.

(5, BFUHS May 2018)

Or

Write a short note on clinicoradiological appearance of giant cell tumor. *(3, DU)*

Or

Write short note on osteoclastoma. *(3, DU)*

Ans: Giant cell tumor or osteoclastoma is a locally aggressive osteolytic tumor of unknown origin.

Etiology: Uncertain.

Age group: 20 to 40 years with female predominance.

Site of involvement

- Epiphyseal end of long bones.
- Distal femur > proximal tibia > distal end of radius.

Clinical features

- Pain is the most common symptom.
- Swelling is another presenting sign. Swelling is eccentrically located over the end of long bones, smooth surface, with normal overlying temperature, may give a sensation of "egg shell cracking" on palpation. Mild to moderate tenderness may be present.
- 10 to 30% cases present with fracture.

Investigations
Radiological

- Well defined single, eccentric located lesion in the subchondral area of the bone.
- There is expansion of the overlying cortex with trabeculae passing through the substance (soap bubble appearance).
- It does not extend into the joint.
- There is no calcification in tumor substance, minimal or no sclerosis around the margins and no new bone formation.

MRI scan

- To define the extent of lesion in bone and soft tissue
- Helps in surgical planning.
- Tumor is dark (hypointense) on T_1-weighted images and bright on T_2-weighted images.

Biopsy: To confirm the diagnosis.

Pathology
Gross

Tumor is eccentrically located in the bone. It is greyish in appearance with loculations and is soft and friable inside.

Microscopic features

There are mononuclear spindle cells interspread with multinucleated giant cells. Giant cells have appearance similar to osteoclasts (bone forming cells). They have multiple nuclei ranging from 50 to 100.

Treatment

1. *Curettage:* A large window is created in the bone overlying tumor and tumor is taken out through that window. The cavity is cleaned with large amount of normal saline to remove any residual tumor.
2. *Curettage with use of adjuvants*
   - Simple curettage had high chances of recurrence due to possibility of residual tumor cells.

- Adjuvants like liquid nitrogen or hydrogen peroxide or phenol or thermal cautery or bone cement (polymethylmethacrylate) is used to clean the cavity after curettage. The adjuvants help in killing the residual tumor cells.

3. *Curettage with bone grafting:* A large defect is created in the bone after curettage. This gap is a stress riser and can lead to fracture of the bone. So, the bone cavity is filled with bone graft taken from patient's own body (autologous) or cadaver (allograft). Sometimes artificial bone graft substitutes or bone cement may also be used to fill the cavity.

4. *Resection only:* In cases where the resection (or complete removal) of tumor shall not result in any major morbidity or loss of function of that body part then excision is also a choice. GCT of proximal end of fibula and distal of ulna are some the examples of the same.

5. *Resection with reconstruction:* In cases where resection-only shall result in significant morbidity or loss of function, the reconstruction is carried out.

   - Arthrodesis (fusion of joint)
     - *Turn-o-plasty:* In this procedure, the tumor is excised and then either tibia or femur is split into half and one and a half is taken turning it upside down and filled in the gap left over. It fixed to the residual bone with screws.
     - *Intercalary fibula grafting:* The gap left after excising the tumor is filled with fibula taken from the lower limb of the same or opposite side.

   - *Arthroplasty (replacement of joint):* In certain cases where there is extension of the tumor into the joint, the lesion is completely resected and the joint is replaced with artificial joint or endoprosthesis. There are situation where we can use combination of allograft and endoprosthesis or allograft only.

6. *Radiotherapy:* Reserved for areas where excision is not feasible or difficult to remove like spine, pelvis or sacrum.

7. *Amputation:* Indicated in cases of malignant transformation and repeated recurrence.

Prognosis: Good but there are chances of recurrence.

Q3. Write a short note on osteochondroma.

(5, *BFUHS May 2010, BFUHS November 2013*)

Or

Describe osteochondroma. (5, *RJ January 2013*)

Ans: It is the most common benign tumor of bone.

Etiopathogenesis

• It is not truly a tumor but developmental malformation. A few peripheral cells from epiphysis grow separately to from a stalk of bone. The growth of bone is faster than this outgrowth hence it lags behind to show up in metaphyseal region. The growth of the bony outgrowth stops at maturity.

• In some cases there is hereditary etiology which results in formation of multiple osteochondromas over the body (hereditary multiple exostosis).

Age group: Patients under the age of 20 years.

Site of involvement

• Metaphyseal region of the bone.

• Distal femur > proximal tibia > proximal humerus

Types

• Pedunculated

• Sessile or broad based

Clinical features

• Painless bony hard palpable swelling.

• Majority of the times it is discovered incidentally.

• Sometimes it may present with pain in cases of
  – Bursitis over the tip of the outgrowth

- Irritation of the adjacent soft tissue
- Fracture through the outgrowth
- Malignant transformation (which may occur in less than 1% cases and rapid growth in size of the swelling in a sign of the same).

Investigations

Radiography: Mature cortical bony outgrowth in the metaphyseal region. It is sufficient to make diagnosis and usually no other investigation is required.

MRI: Required in some cases to look for malignant transformation and to assess the size of cartilaginous cap over the bony outgrowth.

Biopsy: Generally the mass is excised in toto and microscopic examination is carried out.

Pathology

Gross examination: The bony outgrowth has cortex and well differentiated marrow cavity with communication to the marrow cavity of long bone.

Microscopic examination: The cartilaginous cap has appearance similar to normal growth plate but is less well organized. The trabecula inside the cap is formed by endochondral calcification with central core of calcified cartilage.

Treatment

- Majority of the time it is asymptomatic and just requires assurance to the patient that there is no need for any intervention.
- Indications for removal of bony outgrowth are:
  - Pain due to any reason mentioned above under clinical features.
  - Compression of the adjacent neurovascular bundle.
  - Mechanical block to the movement of adjacent joint.
- The operative treatment is excision of the bony outgrowth along with overlying periosteum as there are chances of recurrence from left over cartilage cells.

Q4. Write a short note on radiological features of osteo-chondroma. (5, BFUHS May 2015)

Ans: It is the most common benign tumor of bone. Radiographs are usually sufficient for diagnosis.

Plain radiographs

- Sessile or pedunculated growth in metaphyseal region projecting away from the epiphysis. There is usually associated metaphyseal broadening.
- Calcium deposition (appears as radiopaque) may be seen in cartilaginous cap in some cases.
- Growths after skeletal maturity, cortical destruction are features of malignant transformation.

Computed tomography

- It delineates medullary continuity of the stalk with parent bone better than plain radiographs.
- It is especially useful in cases of compressive myelopathy (CT myelography), i.e. compression of spinal cord.
- Not helpful in detecting malignant transformation.

Ultrasound

- There is hypoechoic signal of cartilaginous cap differentiating from the underlying bone and superficial muscle/fat.
- It can detect bursitis
- It helps in cases when there is suspicion of venous or arterial thrombosis.

Magnetic resonance imaging

- It is the best modality to assess the size of cartilaginous cap accurately (thus helping in detection of malignant transformation). The cartilage shows low signal intensity on T_1-weighted images and high intensity on T_2-weighted images. The increase in size of the cap by more than 1.5 cm is suggestive of malignant transformation. On administration of intravenous contrast there is enhancement of benign lesion but not cartilaginous cap.

- It helps in assessing the relation of neurovascular structures with osteochondroma.
- It detects the presence of bursitis which is the source of pain in a few cases.

Bone scan

- There is increase in uptake of radioactive molecules during growth phase.
- However, if there is increase in uptake after skeletal maturity then it is suggestive of malignancy.

Q5. Write a short note on osteosarcoma.

(5, BFUHS November 2007, 5, RJ January 2009, 3, DU)

Or

Write a short note on osteogenic sarcoma.

(2.5, RJ January 2015)

Or

Write a short note on osteosarcoma of distal end of femur. (3, DU)

Ans: Osteosarcoma is the second most common tumor of bone after giant cell tumor.

Etiology: Origin is thought to be from primitive mesenchymal osteoblastic cells.

Various risk factors have been postulated as:

- Genetic predisposition: Genetic disorders like Li-Fraumeni (p53 mutation), retinoblastoma, Rothmund-Thompson syndrome, fibrous dysplasia, Paget's disease are associated with increased risk for osteosarcoma.
- Radiation exposure.
- Viral infection: HMV and polyoma.
- Family history: Increased risk among first degree relatives.
- Taller and heavier persons are at higher risk.
- History of any other bone cancer.

Age group: It affects mainly two age groups—adolescent (10 to 20 years) and elderly (>60 years). Males show higher incidence as compared to females.

Site of involvement
- Metaphyseal region
- Distal femur > proximal tibia > proximal humerus.

Clinical features
- Pain is the first and chief complaint in majority of cases.
- Swelling is another common symptom. It is eccentrically located over the end of the long bones, variegated consistency (varies between soft and hard) with warm, shiny and stretched skin overlying the swelling. It is tender on palpation.
- Systemic features like fever, night sweats though rare but are present in some cases.
- Tachypnea or respiratory symptoms may be present (indicates pulmonary metastasis).
- Pathological fracture in some cases.
- Lymphadenopathy and decreased range of motion at the adjacent joint.
- Restriction of movements at the adjacent joint due to mechanical block.
- Neurovascular deficit due to compression by tumor in some cases.

Classification: Based upon etiology and histopathology.

Type according to etiology
- *Primary:* The cause is not known. There are no predisposing factors.
- *Secondary:* Predisposing conditions like Paget's disease, fibrous dysplasia and radiation exposure are present.

Type according to histopathology
- Osteoblastic
- Telengiectatic or osteolytic
- Chondroid
- Fibroblastic

Investigations

Blood investigation: Serum alkaline phosphatase is raised but is not diagnostic. It helps in monitoring the cases for recurrence of tumor after excision.

Radiography

- Irregular destruction of the cortex in the metaphyseal area.
- New bone formation in the matrix of the tumor.
- Lesion is osteolytic in approximately 30% of cases, osteoblastic in 45% of cases and mixed in rest of the cases.
- *Codman's triangle:* There is elevation of the periosteum by growing tumor and formation of new bone underneath it. It occurs at the junction of normal and tumor affected bone.
- *Sunburst appearance:* There is calcification of the blood vessels extending from the center of tumor towards the periphery gives this appearance.

MRI: To assess the intramedullary extent, soft tissue involvement and skip lesions.

CT scan

- Helps in delineating the extent of cortical breach and determine the extent of tumor.
- CT scan of chest is helpful in detecting pulmonary metastasis.

Biopsy: To confirm the diagnosis.

Pathology

Gross examination: Tumor is present in the metaphyseal region with variegated consistency ranging from bony hard to soft and friable.

- On cut section, appearance depends upon the predominant histopathology in the tumor, i.e. yellowish white in osteoblastic, cavitation and hemorrhage in telangiectatic, bluish white in chondroid and white in fibroblastic type of osteosarcoma.

Microscopic examination

- There is formation of osteoid (bone) in variable amount by atypical spindle cells.
- The type of osteosarcoma depends upon the predominant extracellular matrix. In osteoblastic there is predominance of new bone, in telangiectatic blood-filled cavities with necrotic areas are seen, in chondroid cartilage predominates, and fibroblastic shows abundance of fibroblasts.

Treatment

- *Chemotherapy:* Neoadjuvant therapy (chemotherapy is started before surgery and then given after tumor excision) in form of methotrexate, cisplatin and doxorubicin is given.
- *Surgical management*
- *Limb salvage surgery:* The tumor is excised with a safe margin of normal tissue and the resulting defect is reconstructed with tumor prosthesis or autograft or allograft.
- *Amputation:* In cases, where limb salvage is not possible, the amputation of the involved limb is performed by taking the safe margin of normal tissue.

Q6. Write a short note on simple bone cyst.

(5, BFUHS May 2016)

Ans: It is also known as unicameral bone cyst. It is a thin-walled cavity filled with straw-colored fluid.

Etiology: Exact cause is not known

Various theories postulated are:

a. Blockage in drainage of interstitial fluid in a rapidly growing and remodeling area of cancellous bone.

b. Venous obstruction within the bone.

c. Synovial cell rests may be present congenitally which could transform later onto cysts.

d. Trauma to growth plate.

e. Genetic association has also been recently postulated.

Age group: Majority of the cases are between age group of 5 and 15 years.

Site of involvement

- Metaphysis
- Proximal humerus > proximal femur > ilium

Clinical features

- In majority of the cases it is diagnosed incidentally while investigating for other problems.
- It may present with pathological fracture.
- Rarely, it may present with growth disturbance.

Differential diagnosis: Aneurysmal bone cyst

Investigations

Radiography

- Well defined radiolucent lesion in the metaphyseal region.
- Fallen leaf sign seen in a few cases, which is free bony fragment lying within the cavity in cases of fracture associated with cyst.

Pathology

Gross: Single cavity with yellowish clear fluid. In cases with associated fracture the cavity may be filled with blood.

Microscopic: The cavity of simple bone cyst consists of lined by fibroblasts. Deep to this layer is fibrovascular tissue.

Treatment

- *Asymptomatic lesions:* Serial observations with radiographs.
- *Large lesion*
  1. Curettage with or without bone grafting
  2. Injection of methylprednisolone into the lesion.
- *Pathological fracture:* Usually heals spontaneously but may require internal fixation in some cases.

Q7. Write a short note on aneurysmal bone cyst.

(5, BFUHS May 2013, 3, DU)

Ans: It is a benign lesion of bone consisting of cavity filled with blood and fibrous septations.

Etiology: Exact etiology is not known.

Various theories postulated are:

• Idiopathic
• Cyst formation could be in response to local hemorrhage formation.
• Local vascular disturbances
• Chromosomal translocation between chromosome numbers 16 and 17.

Age group

• Majority of the patients are younger than 20 years of age.
• Males are more commonly affected than females.

Site of involvement

Metaphyseal area of long bones (proximal humerus, distal femur and proximal tibia) > posterior vertebral elements > pelvis and scapula.

Clinical features

• Pain
• Palpable expansile swelling
• Tenderness on palpation of involved bone
• Sometimes present with pathological fracture.

Differential diagnosis

• Simple bone cyst
• Chondromyxoid fibroma
• Giant cell tumor
• Chondroblastoma
• Osteoblastoma

Investigations

Radiography: Radiolucent lesion seen in the metaphyseal area of the long bone. The lesion may expand to elevate the periosteum but generally remains confined within a shell.

Computed tomography: It is done preoperatively to define the limits of the lesion.

Magnetic resonance imaging: Demonstrates fluid filled cavities with internal septations.

Pathology

Gross: Cavitary lesion with blood filled cavities and internal septations.

Microscopic

- Hemorrhagic tissue with cavitary spaces separated by fibrous tissue composed of spindle cells, inflammatory cells, and a small percentage of giant cells.
- Osteoid formation with or without osteoblastic rimming may be noted.

Treatment

- Treatment of choice: Curettage and bone grafting, with or without adjuvant therapy.
- Wide resection and reconstruction can be considered for lesions that have destroyed the large parts of metaphyseal bone.
- In the axial skeleton and pelvis, arterial embolization can be considered to minimize intraoperative bleeding.
- Recently, radionuclide ablation, cryotherapy and sclerotherapy have been proposed for its management.

Q8. Write a short note on sunray appearance. (3, DU)

Ans: It is radiographic appearance of an aggressive tumor with secondary periostitis.

Pathogenesis: When there is extensive growth of the lesion, the periosteum does not have enough time to lay down the new layer and there is stretching of Sharpey's fibers perpendicular to the bone. These stretched out fibers ossify to give appearance of sunrays on radiograph. It is seen in the following conditions:

1. Osteosarcoma (most common)
2. Ewing's sarcoma
3. Osteoblastic tumors like prostate and lung cancer.

Q9. Write a short note on differential diagnosis of cystic benign tumor of bone. (3, *DU*)

Ans: Differential diagnosis of cystic benign tumor of bone includes the following:

1. Fibrous dysplasia
2. Osteoblastoma
3. Giant cell tumor
4. Myeloma
5. Aneurysmal bone cyst
6. Chondroblastoma
7. Hyperthyroidism
8. Infection
9. Non-ossifying fibroma
10. Enchondroma

(The mnemonic for above list is **FOG MACHINE**).

Clinical features

- Majority of the times it is accidentally detected on radiographs.
- Pain and localized swelling.
- Rarely, it may present as stress fracture through benign cystic lesion.

Diagnosis

X-ray: Anteroposterior and lateral radiographs of the involved limb can detect well defined lytic lesion.

Biopsy: It helps in ascertaining the accurate pathology.

Treatment

- Majority of the benign lytic bone tumors are treated by curettage.
- Following curettage the cavity is cleaned with phenol, normal saline or hydrogen peroxide.
- Subsequently the cavity is filled by autograft, allograft or polymethylmethacrylate (PMMA) (bone) cement.

Chapter 9

Congenital Disorders

Q1. Write a short note on pathology of CTEV.

(5, BFUHS May 2010)

Or

Write a short note on surgical treatment of CTEV.

(5, BFUHS May 2015)

Or

Write a short note on congenital talipes equinovarus.

(3, DU, 3, DU, 5, RJ January 2012)

Or

Write a short note on surgical treatment of club foot.

(3, DU)

Or

Write a short note on deformities in congenital talipes equinovarus. *(3, DU)*

Ans: Incidence

- Overall incidence 1:1,000, though some populations 1:250
- Most common musculoskeletal birth defect
- Male:female ratio approximately 2:1
- It is bilateral in 50% cases.

Pathophysiology: The pathophysiological changes in club foot are as follows:

1. Muscle contractures contributing to the characteristic deformity that include:

- Cavus (tight intrinsic, flexor hallucis longus, flexor digitorum longus)
- Adductus of forefoot (tight tibialis posterior)
- Varus (tight tendo-Achillis, tibialis posterior, tibialis anterior)
- Equinus (tight tendo-Achillis)

2. Bony deformity consists of medial spin of the midfoot and forefoot relative to the hindfoot.
   - Talar neck is medially and plantarly deviated.
   - Calcaneus is in varus and rotated medially around talus
   - Navicular and cuboid are displaced medially.
3. Anterior tibial artery hypoplasia or absence is commonly found in clubfoot.

Genetics
- Genetic component is strongly suggested
- Unaffected parents with affected child have 2.5–6.5% chance of having another child with a clubfoot
- Familial occurrence in 25%

Associated conditions
- Arthrogryposis
- Diastrophic dysplasia
- Myelodysplasia
- Tibial hemimelia
- Amniotic band syndrome (Streeter dysplasia)
- Pierre Robin syndrome
- Larsen syndrome
- Prune-belly syndrome

Clinical features
- Small foot and calf
- Shortened tibia
- Medial and posterior foot skin creases
- Midfoot in cavus
- Forefoot in adduction
- Foot deformities of hindfoot equinus and varus.

These deformities can be differentiated from positional foot deformities by rigid equinus and resistance to passive correction.

Investigations: The diagnosis of clubfoot is mainly clinical. Sometimes radiographs are carried out to document correction in selected cases.

- X-ray of foot
- Anteroposterior view shows talocalcaneal angle (angle between the long axis of talus and calcaneum) is less than 20°.
- Lateral view of foot shows talocalcaneal angle (angle between the long axis of talus and calcaneum) is less than 25°.
- Ultrasonography can detect the clubfoot deformity during pregnancy.

Treatment

- *Non-operative:* It is the most commonly used treatment modality. Ponseti method of serial manipulation and casting and is considered gold standard. French method of daily physical therapy, manipulation and splinting is another method of treatment.
- *Operative:* Rarely used nowadays
  - Posteromedial soft tissue release and tendon lengthening:
    - Indications:
      a. Resistant and/or recurrent feet in young children which could not be cured with Ponseti casting technique.
      b. Clubfoot associated with syndromes like Larsen syndrome, Pierre Robin syndrome, Larsen syndrome, prune-belly syndrome.
      c. Rarely in cases presenting late (e.g. after one year of age)
  - Medial column lengthening or lateral column-shortening osteotomy, or cuboid decancellation.

- Indication: Children presenting at the age of 2 to 3 years
  - Talectomy: It is the removal of talus (a bone in foot)
    - Indications:
      a. Syndrome related clubfoot like arthrogryposis multiplex congenita.
      b. Children presenting at the age of 6 to 10 years
  - Ring fixator application and gradual correction:
    - Indications: Complex deformity resistant to other methods of treatment
    - There are high chances of recurrence after removal of external fixator.
  - Triple arthrodesis: It is fusion of three joints of foot, i.e. calcaneocuboid, talonavicular and subtalar joints.
    - Indication: The child presenting late at age of 10 to 12 years.

Q2. Write a short note on Ponseti technique (3, DU)

Ans: Ponseti technique was developed by Ignacio V. Ponseti for treating congenital clubfoot in the 1940s.

Sequence of correction and methodology by Ponseti technique is as follows:

1. Correction of cavus: Cavus deformity is the first deformity to be corrected.

   Technique

   Forefoot is supinated and the first metatarsal is dorsiflexed. It corrects the forefoot pronation.

2. Correction of adduction and heel varus: Talus is rotated laterally so that the foot abducts underneath the talus leading to lateral rotation of navicular, together with cuboid and anterior aspect of calcaneus, without pronation of foot.

Technique

- The thumb is paced over the head of talus and pressure is applied which lead to abduction and supination of foot. The heel should not be manipulated.
- Cast is applied with adequate padding from toe to groin with knee flexed at 90°.

3. Correction of equinus: Equinus is the last deformity to be corrected.

Technique

- The foot is dorsiflexed after adequate abduction and supination is achieved at foot.
- The foot should not be dorsiflexed prior to correction of hindfoot varus which can lead to rocker bottom foot.
- Percutaneous tenotomy of the Achillis tendon is carried usually before the application of last cast in order to achieve the full correction.

Complications

- Rocker-bottom foot deformity.
- Stiff foot
- Recurrence of deformity.

Q3. Write a short note on congenital dislocation of hip.

(3, DU)

Ans: Incidence

- It is the most common orthopedic disorder in newborns
- More common in females
- bilateral in 20% cases

Risk factors

- Firstborn child
- Female
- Breech delivery

- Family history of congenital dislocation of hip
- Oligohydramnios

Pathophysiology
- There is inherent instability in hip joint due to:
  - Maternal and fetal laxity
  - Genetic laxity
  - Intrauterine and postnatal malpositioning
- The inherent instability in hip leads to dysplasia of femoral hip which leads to gradual dislocation.
- There are associated conditions with it are as:
  - Congenital muscular torticollis
  - Metatarsus adductus
  - Congenital knee dislocation

Clinical features
- The femoral head can be palpated in the posterior aspect of hip
- Limitations in abduction of hip
- *Galeazzi test*
  - There is leg discrepancy with shortening of lower limb on the involved side.
  - When hip is flexed to 90° with feet together, the knee of the involved side is at the lower level than the uninvolved side.
- *Barlow test*: The hip is flexed and adducted. A push is given along the shaft of femur leading to dislocation of the involved hip joint and hence confirms the diagnosis.
- Ortolani's test: The hip is flexed at hip and knee joint to 90°. The thigh is then gently abducted and bringing femoral head from dislocated position into hip joint. The audible can be heard at this stage which confirms the reduction of hip joint.
- *Trendelenburg gait*: The gait is due to abductor insufficiency.

Investigations

- *Radiographs*
    - Anteroposterior view of hip shows:
        a. *Hilgenreiner's line:* A horizontal line is drawn across the both left and right triradiate cartilage. Dislocated femoral head ossification center is superior to this line.
        b. *Perkin's line:* A line perpendicular to the Hilgenreiner's line is drawn to the lateral margin of the acetabulum. Dislocated femoral head is lateral to this line.
        c. *Shenton's line:* It extends across arc along the inferior border of femoral neck and superior margin of obturator foramen. The arc is broken in dislocated hip.
        d. *Acetabular index:* It is the angle between a line drawn from a point on the lateral triradiate cartilage to point on lateral margin of acetabulum and Hilgenreiners line. It is generally greater than 25° in congenital dislocation of hip due to hip dysplasia.
        e. *Center-edge angle (CEA) of Wiberg:* The angle formed by a vertical line from the center of the femoral head and a line from the center of the femoral head to the lateral edge of the acetabulum. It is less than 20° in cases of hip dysplasia.

- **Ultrasonography**
    - It is carried out onto evaluate for acetabular dysplasia and asses for the presence of a hip dislocation.
    - Alpha and beta angles are measured to document the hip dysplasia.

- **Arthrogram**
    - It is injection of dye in the hip joint.
    - Used to confirm the reduction of hip joint after closed maneuver.

- **MRI:** It can used to assess the reduction of hip joint after closed treatment.

Treatment

- *Non-operative*
    a. Abduction brace or pelvic harness:
        – Indication: Children with less than six months
        – Contraindication: In patients with weak hip abductors like in cases of spina bifida or spasticity.
    b. Closed reduction and hip spica application:
        i. Child presenting between six to eighteen months.
        ii. Failure of pelvic harness treatment.
- *Operative*
    a. Open reduction of hip joint and spica application:
        i. Failure of closed reduction
        ii. Child presenting after the age of 18 months.
    b. Open reduction of hip joint and femoral osteotomy:
        i. Children presenting with age between two to four years.
        ii. Femoral head should be congruently reduced.
    c. Open reduction of hip joint and pelvic osteotomy:
        i. Children with age greater than four years
        ii. High acetabular index which denotes acetabular dysplasia.

Chapter 10

Metabolic Bone Disorders

Q1. Write a short note on osteomalacia.

(5, BFUHS November 2008, 3, DU, 3, DU)

Ans: Osteomalacia is a metabolic bone disease where defective mineralization results in a large amount of unmineralized osteoid.

Etiology: Osteomalacia is associated with following conditions:

• Vitamin D deficiency

• Malabsorption syndrome like celiac disease

• Renal osteodystrophy

• Hypophosphatemia

• Chronic alcoholism

• Tumor associated osteomalacia like in parathyroidoma

• Drugs like phenytoin, phenobarbital, rifampin, glucocorticoids.

Symptoms

• Generalized bone and muscle pain. The pain is usually worse at night and rarely relieved by rest.

• Fractures of long bones

• Proximal muscle weakness leading to waddling gait.

Diagnosis

X-ray: Insufficiency fractures are seen in pubic rami, scapula and medial femoral cortex.

Bone scan: Increased activity on triple phase scan.

Blood tests

- Serum calcium is low
- Serum phosphate is low
- Serum vitamin D level is low
- Serum alkaline phosphatase is high
- Serum PTH is high

Treatment

- Treat the underlying problem
- Large doses of oral vitamin D (1000 IU/day).

Q2. Write a short note on treatment of osteoporosis.

(5, BFUHS November 2017)

Ans: Osteoporosis is a bone disease in which mineralization of bony matrix is hampered. This is in contrast to osteomalacia where formation of bony matrix is impaired. Osteoporosis can occur in people of any age, but it is more common in older adults, especially women. People with osteoporosis are at a high risk of fractures, or bone breaks, while doing routine activities.

- Most commonly affected areas are:
  - Proximal femur
  - Distal radius
  - Proximal humerus
  - Spine
- Signs and symptoms:

  Majority of the people do not experience any symptom until they experience fracture. Some features appear in some patients such as:
  - Weak and brittle nails
  - Receding gums
  - Decreased grip strength

In cases of severe osteoporosis, the patient experience fracture of neck of femur, distal end of radius, etc. on trivial fall.

Risk factors for osteoporosis

- Age: After the age of 30 years, the bones tend to break faster than they are replaced and hence are more prone to fracture.
- Menopause: The bone density decreases after the menopause.
- Medical conditions or medications:
  - Hyperthyroidism
  - Hypothyroidism
  - Prednisone or cortisone
- Family history of osteoporosis
- Poor nutrition
- Physical inactivity
- Smoking
- Taking certain medications

Diagnosis

Bone densitometry, or dual-energy X-ray absorptiometry (DEXA). It uses X-rays to measure the density of the bones in your wrists, hips, or spine.

Treatment

- Increase your intake of calcium and vitamin D
- Weight-bearing exercises.
- Bisphosphonates are used to prevent the loss of bone mass. They may be taken orally or by injection. They include:
  - Alendronate
  - Ibandronate
  - Zoledronic acid
- *Hormone therapy*
  - In females, hormonal replacement therapy after menopause helps in reducing bone loss.
  - In males, testosterone therapy may help increase bone density.

- *Raloxifene:* This medication has been found to provide the benefits of estrogen without many of the risks, although there is still an increased risk of deep vein thrombosis.
- *Denosumab:* This drug is taken by injection and may prove even more promising than bisphosphonates at reducing bone loss.
- *Teriparatide:* This drug is also taken by injection and stimulates bone growth.
- *Calcitonin nasal spray:* It is taken as a nasal spray and reduces bone reabsorption. Because osteoporosis medications can have side effects, you may prefer to try other treatments instead of medication.

Osteoporosis prevention

- Taking calcium and vitamin in adequate amount daily.
- Doing weight-bearing exercises
- Stopping smoking
- Hormone replacement therapy in postmenopausal women.

Q3. Write a short note on meniscal injuries.

(5, BFUHS May 2007)

Ans: Menisci are cushions which compensate for incongruity between articulating tibial and femoral condyles.

There are two menisci in knee joints:

- Medial meniscus
- Lateral meniscus

Mechanism of injury: When there is twisting movement of thigh over fixed leg in semi-flexed position, the meniscus is trapped between the femoral and tibial condyles leading to tear along its body. Medial meniscus is more frequently injured because it is less mobile than lateral meniscus.

Classification of meniscal tears

Depending upon the anatomical location:

- Longitudinal tears
- Horizontal tears

- Combination of above two
- Bucket handle tear

Depending upon the zones of vascularity

- *Red zone:* When tear is in the peripheral area at the capsulomeniscal junction
- *Red-white:* Tear at the junction of vascular and less vascular zone
- *White:* When tear is in the less vascular zone

Clinical features

Symptoms

- There is history of injury to knee while playing contact sports.
- Swelling over the knee is present
- Sometimes history of locking while walking or running is present.

Signs

- Tenderness over the medial joint line
- *McMurrays's test:* The knee is flexed and leg is rotated either externally (to check for medial meniscus) or internally (to check for lateral meniscus). It is then slowly extending looking for clicking sound or pain.
- *Apley's grinding test:* The patient is put in prone position. One hand is kept over the back of thigh and with other hand axial compression is given along the long axis of tibia and simultaneously it is rotated internally and externally. Pain on lateral rotation suggests medial meniscus tear and pain on medial rotation suggests lateral meniscus tear.

Diagnosis

X-ray: It cannot detect the meniscal injury but associated bone injuries can be documented.

MRI: It is best investigation to diagnose meniscal tears and other associated ligament injuries.

Arthrography: It can detect tears in meniscus but no longer used due to its invasive nature.

Treatment

• Small tears along the red or red-white zone heals by itself with rest in 3 to 4 weeks.

• Large and chronic tears require surgery in form of arthroscopy. The tears present at the red or red-white zone can sometimes be repaired with sutures while other requires excision.

Q4. Write a short note on rheumatoid factor.

(5, BFUHS May 2013)

Ans: Rheumatoid factor (RF) measures the amount of the antibodies against the Fc fragment of immunoglobulin IgG (rheumatoid factor). It is commonly used in diagnosis of rheumatoid arthritis however; it is not a specific test. The higher levels in a diagnosed case of rheumatoid arthritis are associated with higher chances of disease progression, nodule formation and disease activity.

Generation of RF: IgM autoantibodies are formed against the Fc fragment of immunoglobulin G (IgG). These antibodies then join the normal synovial tissue and various other tissues leading to destruction of joint space and causing joint swelling. It is mainly formed in rheumatoid arthritis however it is seen in many other diseases.

Conduct of test

Latex agglutination test: The blood of patient is mixed with latex beads coated with antibodies. If RF is present it leads to clumping together of latex beads. The amount of agglutination/clumping depends upon the quantity of RF in the blood.

Normal range is below 15 IU/mL.

High levels of RF are seen in following conditions:

• Rheumatoid arthritis

• Autoimmune diseases like SLE, scleroderma, Sjogren's syndrome.

- Liver diseases like cirrhosis, hepatitis
- Infections like tuberculosis, malaria
- Leukemia
- Endocarditis

Falsely elevated RF levels are seen in:
- Fatty individuals
- Elderly more than 65 years
- Multiple blood transfusions

Q5. Write a short note on fluorosis. *(1, RJ January 2009)*

Ans: There is excessive deposition of calcium occurs in bone and soft tissue in fluorosis. It is endemic some parts of Punjab and Andhra Pradesh.

Etiology
- Excessive fluoride intake from drinking water
- Use of coal as a domestic fuel
- Inhalation of fluoride dust in factories

Pathology: The excessive intake of fluorine leads to osteoblastic stimulation. The fluorine compounds are deposited in bone and soft tissue which is resistant to osteoclastic resorption. The tensile strength of bone is reduced.

Clinical features

Dental fluorosis: There is mottling of the dental enamel involving upper incisors especially.

Skeletal fluorosis
- Stiffness of joints
- Restriction of movement at joints
- Paresthesia due to nerve compression by osteo-sclerosis of vertebral bodies
- Extensive vertebral column involvement can present with paraparesis.

Diagnosis
- Blood tests:
  - Mild to moderate anemia
  - Raised fluoride levels in blood

– Fluoride levels are raised in urine
– X-ray shows extensive calcification in vertebrae, sacroiliac ligaments, interosseous membrane.

Treatment
• Decrease the intake of fluoride
• Chemical defluoridation (Nalgonda technique)
• Avoid fluoride toothpastes.

Q6. Write a short note on gout. *(1, RJ January 2011)*

Ans: It is a hereditary disorder characterized by disorder of purine metabolism affecting middle-aged males and postmenopausal females.

Etiology: The exact cause is not known however there are predisposing factors which have been implicated:
• Alcoholism
• Obesity
• Hemolytic disorder
• High dietary intake of purine-rich diet like meats, beans, pulses, lentils.
• Long-term use of diuretics

Pathogenesis
The blood uric acid levels in body may be due to either of following reasons:
• *Undersecretion of uric acid:* Patients taking diuretics, aspirin, ethambutol, pyrazinamide, etc.
• *Overproduction of uric acid:* Patients with diseases like lymphomas, leukemias, etc.
• *Both undersecretion and overproduction:* High intake of alcohol and obesity.

There is deposition of monosodium urate crystals (also known as tophi) in synovium of joints due to high serum uric acid levels. There is breakage of these crystals whenever there is fluctuation of uric acid levels in the body. The crystals are ingested by macrophages which initiate a chronic inflammatory reaction in the joints and hence joint destruction. Many times it is seen that high uric acid level does not lead to gout so it is the fluctuations in the serum uric acid levels which precipitate a gouty attack.

Clinical features

Acute gout: Severe pain with localized swelling and redness. Most commonly great toe is involved while small joints of hands, elbow and knee may be involved. *Chronic gout:* There are formation of nodules (tophi described earlier) around the small joints of hand or feet. There severe destruction of large joints like knee and elbow presenting with stiffness and deformity.

Diagnosis

Blood tests: Serum uric acid levels may or may not be raised.

X-ray

- Soft tissue swelling
- Punched out lesion with overhanging bony edges (G-sign).
- Joint space narrowing with deformity seen in advanced stages.

Joint aspiration: The joint is aspirated and subjected to microscopic examination. The presence of strongly negative birefringent needle shaped crystals are suggestive of gout.

Treatment

- *Asymptomatic hyperuricemia:* No treatment required
- *Acute gout*
  - Rest and ice application over the joint
  - Non-steroidal anti-inflammatory drugs are given
  - Colchicine can lower the uric acid levels
  - Corticosteroids: Decrease the swelling
- *Chronic gout*
  - Low purine diet
  - Allopurinol
  - Febuxostat
  - Non-steroidal anti-inflammatory drugs
  - Probenecid for underexcretors

Q7. Write a short note on rickets.

(5, BFUHS May 2012, November 2012)

Ans: Definition: There is defect in mineralization of osteoid matrix by inadequate calcium and phosphate deposition prior to physeal closure.

Pathophysiology

- There is disturbance of calcium and phosphate metabolism.
- Poor calcium deposition at zone of provisional calcification (which is the growing end of long bones) leading to widening of physis, cortical thinning and bowing.

Radiographic findings

- Genu varum and valgum
- Decreased bone density
- Looser's zone: Pseudofracture on the compression side of bone
- Physeal widening
- Metaphyseal cupping

Laboratory diagnosis

Disease	Serum calcium	Serum phosphate	Serum alkaline phosphatase	Serum PTH	Serum vitamin D
Vitamin D deficit	Low	Low	High	High	Low
Vitamin D-dependent	Low	Low	High	High	Normal to low
Vitamin D-resistant	Normal to low	Low	High	High	Normal to low
Renal osteodystrophy	Low	High	high	High	Normal
Hypophosphatasia	High	High	Low	Normal to low	Normal to low

Classification
- Vitamin D deficient
- Vitamin D dependent
- Vitamin D resistant
- Renal osteodystrophy
- Hypophosphatasia
- Vitamin D deficiency rickets (nutritional)

Etiology: Nutritional rickets is associated with decreased dietary intake of vitamin D. It is commonly seen in:
- Premature infants
- Malabsorption syndrome (celiac sprue) or chronic parental nutrition.

Clinical features
- Bowing of knees
- Rachitic rosary
- Waddling gait
- Codfish vertebrae
- Muscular hypotonia
- Dental disease

Treatment
- Vitamin D 5000 IU daily till vitamin D levels are normal.

  Vitamin D-dependent rickets
  - Pathophysiology: It is of two types:

    a. *Type I:* Defect in enzyme 25α-hydroxylase

    b. *Type II:* Defect in intracellular receptor for 1,25-hydroxyvitamin D.

Clinical features
- Multiple joints pain
- Muscle hypotonia
- Growth retardation

- Hypocalcemic seizures
- Fractures in early infancy

Laboratory diagnosis: Type II is distinguished from type I by markedly elevated levels of 1,25-(OH) 2-vitamin D.

Treatment

- Daily 1 μm/day of 1,25-(OH)2-vitamin D
- Daily high dose vitamin D and calcium

Vitamin D-resistant rickets

Etiology: There is inability of renal tubules to absorb phosphate. It has X-linked dominant inheritance.

Clinical features: They are similar to vitamin D deficient rickets.

Treatment: Vitamin D along with phosphate supplementation.

Q8. Describe radiological features of rickets.

*(2, RJ January 2013, 1,
RJ January 2011, 1, RJ January 2009)*

Ans: Rickets is characterized by defect in mineralization of osteoid matrix by inadequate calcium and phosphate deposition prior to physeal closure.

Radiological features of rickets are

- Decreased bone density
- *Epiphysis:* There is widened and irregular epiphysis
- *Metaphysis:* Fraying, widening and cupping of the metaphysis.
- Bowing of long bone with genu varum or varum
- *Scoliosis:* Side bending of spine
- *Triradiate pelvis:* There is protrusion of proximal femur into pelvis.
- *Looser's zone:* Pseudofracture on the compression side of bone.

Mnemonic RICKETS

- **R**eaction of the periosteum
- **I**ndistinct cortex

- Coarse trabeculation
- Knees, wrists, and ankles affected predominantly
- Epiphyseal plates, widened and irregular
- Tremendous metaphysis (cupping, fraying, splaying)
- Spur (metaphyseal)

Q9. Write a short note on vitamin D resistant rickets.

(3, DU)

Ans: It is hereditary disorder characterized by resistance to administration of large doses of vitamin D.

Types

1. Hypophosphatemic rickets
2. Pseudo-deficiency rickets

Hypophosphatemic rickets

- It is due to mutation in PHEX (phosphate regulating endopeptidase) gene.
- X-linked dominant
- Treated with phosphates and one hydroxy derivatives of vitamin D.
- Deformities can be prevented with treatment.

Pseudo-deficiency rickets

- There is severe hypocalcemia with hyperparathyroidism
- Autosomal recessive inheritance.
- The child presents with bone deformities, muscular hypotonia, dental anomalies and features of hypocalcemia.
- Laboratory diagnosis:

Disease	Serum calcium	Serum phosphate	Serum alkaline phosphatase	Serum PTH	Serum vitamin D
Vitamin D resistant	Normal to low	Low	High	High	Normal to low

Types

a. *Type I:* Genetic mutation in cytochrome P450: It responds to one hydroxyvitamin D derivative.

b. *Type II:* Genetic mutation in vitamin D receptor: It does not respond to high dose of vitamin D.

Q10. Write a short note on Paget's disease. *(3, DU)*

Ans: It is bone remodeling disorder in which there is excessive bone resorption followed by new bone formation. This leads to large amount of new bone which is weak and prone to fracture.

Incidence

• Peak incidence is in 5th decade of life

• Equally affects males and females

• Common sites of involvement are femur > pelvis > tibia > skull > spine.

Pathology

• Autosomal dominant inheritance

• There are irregular broad trabeculae with large multinucleated osteoclasts. vascular tissue interspersed between trabeculae.

Phases of Paget's disease: It passes through three phases and all the three phases may coexist in same bone.

• *Lytic phase:* There is osteoclastic resorption.

• *Mixed phase:* Resorption and compensatory bone formation.

• *Sclerotic phase:* Bone formation predominates.

Clinical features

• Majority of the times it is incidentally detected

• Pain

• Swelling

• There may be associated cardiac problems like high output cardiac failure.

Diagnosis

- *X-ray:* Depending upon the phase of disease, the presentation may be lucent areas in lytic phase and sclerotic in sclerotic phase. There is loss of distinction between medulla and cortex.
- *CT scan:* There is cortical thickening and coarsening of trabeculae.
- *Bone scan:* The uptake is high in lytic phase and low in sclerotic phase.
- *Blood test:* Serum calcium levels are normal with high serum alkaline phosphatase.
- *Urine examination:* High levels of urinary N-telopeptide and α-C-telopeptide.

Treatment

Non-operative

- Asymptomatic patients require observation only
- Pain is treated with NSAIDs.
- Bisphosphonates inhibit osteoclast and osteoblast activity.
- Calcitonin inhibits osteoclastic activity.

Operative

- Metaphyseal osteotomy in bowed bones
- Joint replacement in arthritic joints.

Q11. Enumerate diagnostic criteria for rheumatoid arthritis. *(3, DU)*

Ans: American College of Rheumatology drafted criteria in 2010 for diagnosis of rheumatoid arthritis. Definite RA is based upon the presence of synovitis in at least one joint, the absence of an alternative diagnosis that better explains the synovitis, and the achievement of a total score of at least 6 (of a possible 10) from the individual scores in four domains. The highest score achieved in a given domain is used for this calculation. These domains and their values are:

1. Number and site of involved joints:
   - 2 to 10 large joints (from among shoulders, elbows, hips, knees, and ankles) = 1 point.
   - 1 to 3 small joints (from among the metacarpophalangeal joints, proximal interphalangeal joints, second through fifth metatarsophalangeal joints, thumb interphalangeal joints, and wrists) = 2 points.
   - 4 to 10 small joints = 3 points
   - Greater than 10 joints (including at least 1 small joint) = 5 points

2. Serological abnormality (rheumatoid factor or anti-citrullinated peptide/protein antibody):
   - Low positive (above the upper limit of normal [ULN]) = 2 points
   - High positive (greater than three times the ULN) = 3 points

3. Elevated acute phase response (erythrocyte sedimentation rate [ESR] or C-reactive protein [CRP]) above the ULN = 1 point.

4. Symptom duration at least six weeks = 1 point.

   In addition to those with the criteria above, which are best suited to patients with newly presenting disease, the following patients are classified as having RA:

   a. Patients with erosive disease typical of RA with a history compatible with prior fulfillment of the criteria above.

   b. Patients with long-standing disease, including those whose disease is inactive (with or without treatment) who have previously fulfilled the criteria above based upon retrospectively available data.

Metabolic Bone Disorders | **131**

Q12. Write a short note on scurvy.

Or

Write clinical features of scurvy. *(2, RJ January 2015)*

Ans: Scurvy is due to vitamin C deficiency.

Incidence
- Common in infants aged between 6 months and 1 year
- It affects wrist, knee and sternal end of ribs
- It is more common in alcoholics, smokers, chronic malnutrition, malabsorption syndrome.

Pathophysiology
- Vitamin C deficiency leads to impaired chondroitin sulfate and collagen synthesis especially collagen type I.
- The intracellular hydroxylation of collagen is absent.
- Deficiency of collagen leads to altered new bone formation.

Clinical features

Symptoms
- Multiple bones pain
- Generalized weakness (pseudoparalysis) and myalgia
- Diarrhea, tachypnea, fever
- Irritability
- There is bleeding from gums, hematuria, hematemesis.

Signs
- Joint effusions
- Petechiae and ecchymosis
- Scorbutic rosary
- Palpable swelling over the subcutaneous bones lie ulna and tibia due to subperiosteal hemorrhage.
- Frog leg posture due to flexion at hip and knee.

- Hypotension in late stages
- Hyperkeratosis is seen in adult scurvy
- Subconjunctival hemorrhages and bleeding gums.

Investigations

Radiography: Anteroposterior and lateral X-rays of wrist and knee reveals

- *White line of Frankel:* Wide zone of provisional calcification.
- *Trummerfeld zone:* It is a radiolucent band of metaphysic adjacent to Frankel line.
- *Wimberger ring*: There is ring of increased density surrounding epiphysis.
- Metaphyseal spurs
- Pencil thin cortex
- Subperiosteal elevation
- Ground glass appearance of metaphysis

Blood test: Serum ascorbic acid level is low.

Treatment

- Treat the cause
- Vitamin C supplementation.

Chapter 11

Soft Tissue Problems

Q1. Write a short note on tennis elbow.

(2, RJ January 2011, 1, RJ January 2009, 3, DU)

Ans: It is also known as lateral epicondylitis.

Etiology: It is thought to occur because of overuse injury to the extensor group of muscles at the elbow (specifically extensor carpi radialis brevis).

Pathophysiology: There is microscopic tearing of the extensor carpi radialis which leads to angiofibroblastic reaction at the lateral epicondyle.

Clinical features

- Pain over the lateral aspect of elbow
- Point tenderness over the lateral epicondyle.
- **Cozen's test:** There is pain over the lateral aspect of elbow on dorsiflexion of wrist against resistance in extension.
- *Mill's test:* There is pain over the lateral aspect of elbow on pronating the forearm in a flexed wrist with extended elbow.
- *Maudsley's test:* There is pain over the lateral aspect of elbow on extending the middle finger with extended elbow.

Investigations

X-ray of the elbow AP and lateral view: It is usually normal except in a few circumstances where there could be calcification over the lateral aspect of elbow.

MRI: It can detect degenerative changes in the origin of the extensor carpi radialis.

Management

Non-operative

- Majority of the cases are treated with this method.
- Nonsteroidal anti-inflammatory drugs (NSAIDs) are the first line of treatment.
- Local steroidal injections are administered if there is no relief with NSAIDs.
- Injection of platelet-rich plasma over the involved area.
- Ultrasonic diathermy.
- Avoid heavy weight lifting.
- Extracorporeal shock wave therapy.
- Extension exercises at the elbow joint.

Operative treatment

- In rare cases when conservative treatment fails.
- The fibrous tissue at the origin of extensor carpi radialis is excised.
- Percutaneous release at the lateral epicondyle is another option in selected cases.

Q2. Write a short note on frozen shoulder.

(2, RJ January 2016)

Ans: It is also known as adhesive capsulitis or periarthritis shoulder.

Etiology

- Common among elderly females
- Trauma
- Diabetes

- Ischemic heart disease
- Hypothyroidism
- Systemic inflammatory diseases

Pathology: There is fibroblastic proliferation of the shoulder joint capsule which results in adhesion formation and hence stiffness at the shoulder joint.

Clinical features

- Pain on shoulder movements
- Restriction of movement at the involved shoulder joint especially external rotation and abduction.

Stages of frozen shoulder

The frozen shoulder passes through three phases:

1. *Painful phase:* There is pain in the involved shoulder
2. *Phase of stiffening:* There is restriction of movement at the shoulder joint.
3. *Resolution phase:* There is restoration of movements at the shoulder joint.

Investigations

X-ray: There is no abnormality seen on the radiographs.

MRI: It is carried out to rule out any associated rotator cuff pathology.

Treatment

- The disease is chiefly self-limiting. It is resolves with time.
- NSAIDs are given to counter the pain.
- Physiotherapy in form of range of motion exercises at the shoulder joint are advised.
- Manipulation under anesthesia is done in selected cases to increase the range of movement.
- In resistant cases: Open or arthroscopic release is carried out to achieve the movement at the shoulder joint.

Q3. Write a short note on trigger finger.

(5, BFUHS May 2011)

Or

Write a short note on trigger thumb.

(1, RJ January 2008)

Ans: Definition: It is also known as stenosing tenosynovitis. In this condition the finger is stuck in bent position and on straightening the finger there is snap.

Etiology

- Exact etiology is unknown
- Higher incidence is seen in patients with:
  - Diabetes mellitus
  - Autoimmune disorders like psoriatic arthritis, rheumatoid arthritis, sarcoidosis.
  - Secondary infection like tuberculosis

Pathophysiology: There is inflammation of the tendon sheath which surrounds the tendon. The inflammation is followed by formation of nodule in sheath. Normally the tendon passes under narrow pulleys (like a train passing through narrow subway) and due to formation of nodule it not able to pass under the pulleys smoothly, hence leading to triggering of finger.

Clinical features

- Most commonly the middle and ring fingers are involved
- There is painful clicking as the finger is moved through flexion and extension.
- There is palpable tender nodule over the metacarpal head.

Differential diagnosis

- Rheumatoid arthritis
- Ganglion involving the tendon sheath
- Dupuytren's contracture
- Acromegaly may lead to deposition of extracellular matrix in tendon sheath leading to trigger finger.

Investigations

- It is a clinical diagnosis
- If there is concern about uncontrolled associated diabetes mellitus and rheumatoid arthritis then HbA1c and rheumatoid factor can be tested.
- Radiographs can be done to exclude osteoarthritis, fracture malunion or a foreign body that is affecting interphalangeal joint motion.

Treatment: The various treatment options for trigger finger include:

- Orthoses (splinting)
- Corticosteroid injections
- Corticosteroid injections along with use of orthoses
- Surgery: The transverse incision is given over the tendon nodule and A2 pulley is incised.

Q4. Write a short note on painful arc syndrome.

(5, RJ January 2016)

Ans: Painful arc syndrome or impingement syndrome is characterized by pain referred to the lateral aspect of the upper arm in the region of deltoid muscle.

Pathology: Rotator cuff impingement passes through three stages:

- *Stage 1*
  - It affects patient younger than 25 years
  - Characterized by edema, inflammation and hemorrhage in the rotator cuff.
  - Reversible in nature and can be treated non-operatively.
- *Stage 2*
  - It affects patient aged between 25 and 40 years
  - Characterized by fibrosis and tendinitis in rotator cuff.
  - Non-reversible in nature and generally requires operative intervention.

- *Stage 3*
  - It affects patient aged older than 40 years
  - Characterized by disruption of fibers of rotator cuff and osteophytes from the acromion
  - Irreversible in nature and requires operative intervention.

Clinical features

- The pain is characteristic in specific arc (30° to 120°) of shoulder motion.
- Sharp pain in the shoulder especially on overhead activities and at night time.
- Deltoid muscle wasting in long-standing cases.
- Limitation of range of motion at shoulder joint.
- There is progressive weakness in the strength of the shoulder joint.
- Tests for impingement:
  - *Neer test:* On forward elevation and internal rotation of arm there is pain in shoulder.
  - *Hawkin's test:* Forceful internal rotation of a 90° forwardly flexed arm leads to pain.
  - *Impingement test:* Injection of 1 mL of 10% xylocaine into subacromial space leads to resolution of symptoms.

Diagnosis

X-ray: Anteroposterior and lateral radiograph of shoulder can detects features like osteophytes from acromion and signs of instability like Hill-Sachs lesion.

MRI: It can accurately identify lesions in rotator cuff.

Treatment

Non-operative

- Range of motion and strengthening exercises at shoulder joint
- Nonsteroidal anti-inflammatory drugs
- Cortisone injections.

Operative

• When patient does not respond to non-operative treatment.

• Open or arthroscopic removal of osteophytes from acromion with rotator cuff repair if required.

Q5. Write a short note on Dupuytren's contracture.

(3, DU)

Ans: There is fibrous metaplasia of the subcutaneous tissue of palm.

Etiology: The exact pathology is not known. The predisposing factors have been described as follows:

1. Diabetes

2. Alcoholism

3. Smoker

4. Antiepileptic drugs

5. Manual laborers

6. Ledderhose's disease (fibrous of medial plantar fascia)

Clinical features

• Bilateral in 50% cases

• Palpable nodules are present at the base of fingers

• There is flexion contracture at the metacarpophalangeal and interphalangeal contracture joints in long-standing cases.

Pathology: The palmar fascia is replaced with fibrous tissue in the form of nodule and cords. There is subsequently secondary contracture resulting in flexion contractures at the joints. Ring finger is most commonly involved in it.

Treatment

1. No treatment is required for minimal deformity.

2. Total or partial fasciectomy: Partial or total removal of palmar fascia. It is indicated when flexion contracture is more than 15° at proximal interphalangeal joint and 30° at metacarpophalangeal joint.

3. Rarely amputation is indicated when there is recurrence of contracture after surgery or in severe cases.

Q6. Write a short note on carpal tunnel syndrome.

(5, BFUHS November 2006, 1, RJ January 2012, 3, DU)

Ans: It is a compressive neuropathy in which there is compression of median nerve at the carpal tunnel.

Etiopathogenesis: There is no single etiology for carpal tunnel syndrome. Various risk factors have been implicated as follows:

1. Obesity

2. Pregnancy

3. Female

4. Hypothyroidism

5. Rheumatoid arthritis

6. Smoking

7. Alcoholism

8. Chronic renal failure

9. Space occupying lesions like ganglion, neuroma.

Clinical features

- Pain and paresthesia over the lateral half of the palm and three fingers.
- Pain in more severe in night due to flexion at the wrist leading to decrease space in carpal tunnel syndrome
- *Phalen test:* Acute flexion at wrist for more than 60 seconds leads to paresthesia in hand.
- *Durkan test:* Direct compression of median nerve at carpal tunnel leads to paresthesia in hand.

Diagnosis

- *Nerve conduction velocity:* It shows latency of more than 4.5 milliseconds in median nerve.
- *Electromyography:* It shows positive sharp waves and fibrillations at rest.

- *MRI:* It shows space occupying lesions in the carpal tunnel syndrome.

Treatment

Non-operative

- Night splint to prevent wrist flexion.
- Corticosteroids injection in the carpal tunnel to relieve symptoms.

Operative

Indicated in cases not responding to conservative treatment, open or arthroscopic release of carpal tunnel is advised.

Chapter 12

Miscellaneous Bone Diseases

Q1. Write a short note on triple arthrodesis.

(5, BFUHS November 2006, 5, BFUHS May 2006)

Ans: Definition: It is surgical fusion of three joints of foot, i.e. talocalcaneal, talonavicular and calcaneocuboid.

Goal of the surgery: To achieve painless, plantigrade and stable foot.

Indications for the surgery
- Post-traumatic arthritis
- Tibialis posterior dysfunction
- Tarsal coalition
- Cavus and cavovarus
- Valgus deformities of the foot that cannot be managed with braces.
- Neuromuscular dysfunction.

Contraindications for the surgery
- Foot deformities that can be managed with braces
- Chronic smoker
- Children (aged less than 12)

Surgical technique
- Two incisions given over the medial and lateral aspects of the foot.
- The three joints—talocalcaneal, talonavicular and calcaneocuboid are opened up. The cartilage is

removed and resulting bone defects are filled with bone grafts. The joints are then stabilized with hardwares or implants. The foot is placed in plaster till there is complete bony fusion.

Complications

- Non-union at the site of operation
- Local wound complications
- Residual deformity
- Avascular necrosis of the talus
- Ankle and mid-tarsal arthritis

Q2. Write a short note on triple deformity of knee.

(2, RJ January 2015)

Ans: Triple deformity, i.e. valgus, external rotation, flexion deformity of knee with posterior subluxation of tibia.

Etiopathogenesis: It is usually seen in:

- Tuberculosis of knee (most common cause)
- Rheumatoid arthritis
- Post-traumatic incompletely reduced old neglected dislocated knees.

Pathogenesis: In tuberculosis of knee, there is erosion of cartilage which exposes the subchondral bone. When there is progression of disease, there is advancement in bony destruction and joint is filled with granulation or fibrous tissue. There is disruption of knee ligaments and knee joint goes into triple deformity. Initially the spasm of hamstring muscles (primarily biceps femoris) leads to flexion at knee, lateral subluxation and external rotation of tibia. Tensor fascia lata along with iliotibial band further increases the deformity. In long-standing cases, there is contracture of the posterior capsule.

Diagnosis

X-ray: Anteroposterior and lateral view of the knee shows the deformity.

Blood tests: ESR and CRP can detect the infectious pathology like tuberculosis.

Biopsy: It can detect the exact pathology like granuloma formation in tuberculosis and pannus formation in rheumatoid arthritis.

Treatment

- Antitubercular drugs in cases of TB knee
- Disease modifying drugs in case of rheumatoid arthritis.
- Double traction: One in line of tibia and other at right angles to it is given to correct the deformity. Double traction is helps to:
  1. Correct and prevent deformities
  2. Distract articular margins and minimize pain
  3. Relieve muscle spasm
- In advanced and neglected cases, arthrodesis is advised.

Q3. Write a short note on Thomas splint.

(5, BFUHS May 2013)

Ans: Hugh Owen Thomas designed and developed Thomas splint in 1865. It was first developed for treating knee tuberculosis and later used for management of lower limb fractures. It was popularized by his nephew Sir Robert Jones.

Components of Thomas splint

- It consists of a proximal padded oval ring fitted around the groin with ischial tuberosity as a fixed point.
- The ring was attached by two iron rods to a smaller ring below. The inner rod was attached to the proximal ring at an angle of 45°.
- A sheet is stretched across the two bars to support the limb.
- Strapping was applied to the leg and traction was gained by tying this to the cross-bar at the distal end of the splint.
- Pearson attachment: Thomas splint can be attached with Pearson attachment for knee mobilization.

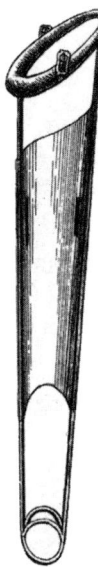

Measurement of length of Thomas splint required

- Ring diameter equal to thigh width in line with inguinal ligament is measured and two inches are added to the measured width.
- The length of splint is measured from the groin to the tip of heel and six inches are added to the measurement.

Uses

- Fractures of lower limb
- Transportation of patients with lower limb injuries
- Immobilization of knee in tuberculosis of knee
- Both skin and skeletal traction can be applied through it.
- Fixed traction can also given through it.

Q4. Mention sites of avascular necrosis.

(1, RJ January 2008)

Ans: Avascular necrosis is commonly seen at following sites:

- Head of femur
- Scaphoid

- Talus
- Lunate
- Head of humerus
- Bisphosphate-induced avascular necrosis of jaw.

Q5. Write a short note on knock knee. (*1, RJ January 2008*)

Or

Write a short note on genu valgum. (*3, DU*)

Ans: Knock knees are condition in which the knees touch, but the ankles do not touch. The legs turn inward.
Site of bony involvement: Distal femur is the most common location followed by tibia.

Etiology

Bilateral genu valgum
- Physiologic
- Renal rickets
- Skeletal dysplasia
- Morquio syndrome

Unilateral genu valgum
- Physeal injury from trauma or infection
- Proximal tibia fracture
- Benign tumors
- Fibrous dysplasia

Physiological knock knees
- At birth, child has genu varum which progresses to genu valgum between 3 and 4 years.
- After the age of seven, the intermalleolar distance should be less than 8 cm

Treatment
Non-operative
- When genu valgum is less than 15° and child is less than 6 years old only observation is required.
- There is no role of bracing

Operative

Hemiepiphysiodesis of medial side.

Indication: Greater than 15° of valgus in a patient aged less than 10 years.

Technique: Staples are applied over the medial aspect of epiphysis to stop its growth while the other side grows normally.

Distal femoral varus osteotomy

- *Indications:* Insufficient remaining growth for hemiepiphysiodesis.

- *Technique:* Closing wedge osteotomy is performed. Special care is taken to prevent injury to peroneal nerve.

Q6. Write a short note on Osgood-Schlatter disease.

(1, RJ January 2008)

Ans: It is traction apophysitis of tibial tubercle.

Incidence

- More common in adolescent males
- It is a self-limiting disease.

Clinical features

- Pain over the anterior aspect of knee which is aggravated by kneeling.
- There is tenderness over the tibial tuberosity
- Swelling over the tibial tuberosity.

Diagnosis

X-ray: Anteroposterior and lateral view of the knee shows irregularity and fragmentation of the tibial tubercle.

MRI: There is irregularity and fragmentation of tibial tubercle.

- Soft tissue swelling
- Thickening and edema of patellar tendon

Differential diagnosis

1. Tibial tubercle fractures
2. Osteochondroma
3. Avulsion injury of inferior pole of patella.

Treatment

Non-operative

- Majority of the patients can be managed conservatively.
- Rest, ice application, activity modification and NSAIDs.
- In patients not responding to above treatment, the limb is immobilized in case of 6 weeks.

Operative

- Indicated in skeletally mature refractory cases
- Ossicle is excised as symptomatic relief is achieved.

Q7. Write a short note on housemaid's knee.

(1, RJ January 2009)

Ans: It is also known as prepatellar bursitis, there swelling or inflammation over the anterior aspect of the knee.

Incidence

- Excessive kneeling
- Higher incidence in wrestlers.

Clinical features

- History of repeated kneeling over the knee
- Pain and swelling over the anterior aspect of knee
- Local temperature is raised if there is associated sepsis.

Diagnosis

- It is mainly clinical
- In cases of suspected sepsis, the aspirate is subjected to gram staining.

Treatment

Non-operative: Rest, NSAIDs, aspiration and compression bandage application.

Operative: Open or arthroscopic resection of bursa.

Q8. Write a short note on hallux valgus. (3, DU)

Ans: Hallux valgus is outward deviation of the great toe. It is not an isolated deformity of great toe but associated with symptoms of lesser toes also.

Etiology: No single cause has been identified. There are predisposing factors implicated in its occurrence as follows:

- Females are more prone than males
- Genetic predisposition
- Rheumatoid arthritis
- Pes planus
- Cerebral palsy
- Use of high heel and narrow toe box.

Types

a. Adult

b. Juvenile or adolescent

Pathoanatomy

- Valgus (outward) deviation of the phalanx
- Varus (inward) deviation of the metatarsal head
- Medial part of capsule of 1st MCP joint is stretched while lateral part is contracted.
- Sesamoid bones (small vestigial bones present around the metatarsophalangeal joint of great toe) are displaced medially.

Clinical features

Symptoms

- Difficulty in wearing shoes
- Pain over the medial eminence.

Signs

- Great toe is in attitude of valgus and pronation on examination.
- There is callous formation medially over metatarsophalangeal joint of great toe.
- There are lesser toe deformities.

Radiographs: Anteroposterior, lateral, oblique and weight-bearing X-rays of the feet help in quantification of deformity. The degenerative changes in the small joints of the foot can be noted.

Treatment

Non-operative: Shoe modifications, pads or spacers can be used in cases not willing for operative intervention.

Operative

- McBride procedure
- Modified McBride procedure
- Metatarsal osteotomies
- Phalangeal osteotomies
- Metatarsophalangeal joint arthrodesis
- Proximal phalanx resection arthroplasty.

Q9. Write a short note on hallux rigidus.

(2, RJ January 2013)

Ans: It is a condition characterized by loss of movement at first metatarsophalangeal joint due to degenerative arthritis.

Etiopathogenesis

- Exact reason is not known
- Genetic predisposition has been postulated
- Acute or repetitive microtrauma.

Clinical features

- Pain and swelling over the great toe
- Restriction of dorsiflexion at the MTP joint.

Diagnosis

X-ray: Anteroposterior, lateral and weight-bearing radiographs show osteophytes, joint space narrowing and subchondral cyst formation and sclerosis.

Treatment

Non-operative: NSAIDs, shoe and activity modification.

Operative

- Joint debridement and synovectomy
- Dorsal cheilectomy
- Resection arthroplasty
- MTP joint arthrodesis

Q10. Write a short note on Morant Baker cyst. (3, *DU*)

Ans: Popliteal synovial cysts, also known as Baker's cysts, are commonly found in association with intra-articular knee disorders, such as osteoarthritis and meniscus tears.

Pathology

- There is a valvular opening in capsule on the posterior and deep medial aspect of the gastrocnemius which allows the fluid to pass from knee joint into the cyst and there is only one way communication.
- The wall of cyst is lined by synovial tissue with evident fibrosis. There may be loose bodies seen in the cyst.

Clinical features

- Popliteal swelling
- Pain over the posterior aspect of the knee
- Sometimes mechanical blockade to knee flexion
- Fouchner sign: The cyst will be firm in full knee extension and soft when the knee is flexed.

Differential diagnosis

- Popliteal artery aneurysm
- Soft tissue tumors
- Meniscal cyst
- Hematoma
- Thromboembolism.

Diagnosis

- **X-ray:** Help in detecting associated pathologies commonly associated with popliteal cysts such as osteoarthritis, loose bodies.

- *Arthrogram*: Injection of dye into joint shows communication between joint and cyst.
- *Ultrasound*: The cysts appear anechoic on ultrasound, indicating that they are fluid filled. Echogenic areas, representing loose bodies, may occasionally be seen within a popliteal cyst.
- *MRI*: It is gold standard in diagnosis and helps defining the exact intra-articular pathology.

Complications
- Infection
- Rupture
- Neurovascular compression.

Treatment
Non-operative
- Quadriceps exercises for six weeks
- Intra-articular steroid injection decreases the size of cyst.

Operative
- Surgical excision of the Baker's cyst treatment of any intra-articular lesions.
- Arthroscopic debridement of the cyst.

Q11. Write a short note on tension band wiring.

(1, RJ January 2008)

Ans: When a wiring or plating is done on the tensile surface (outer surface) of the bone, there is compression at the fracture site on flexion and gap on extension. This conversion of tension forces into compressive forces is tension band principle.

Q12. Write a short note on lag screw.

(1, RJ January 2011, 1, RJ January 2009)

Ans: Lag screw technique involves placement of one or more screws across the fracture site to achieve compression between two bony fragments. The direction of compression or lag screw must be perpendicular to the fracture surface.

Q13. Write a short note on Russell traction. (3, DU)

Ans: It is a form of skin traction designed by Hamilton Russell.

Indication: It is used in treatment of femoral shaft fracture in children.

Principle: Application: Adhesive strips are applied over the leg and knee is suspended in a sling. A rope is attached to the sling spreader bar and the rope is attached to a overhead bar and passed over a pulley. The rope is attached to three pulleys at the foot end of bed: First to a pulley on the bed's foot bar, next to a pulley attached to the foot spreader bar, and then back to a second pulley on the bed's foot bar. There is upward pulley by the sling and pull towards the foot the angle between the thigh and bed is 20°.

Advantages
- Cheap and readily available
- Muscle atrophy is minimized and joint motion invariably preserved.
- Management of compound injuries is easy
- Mild malposition is corrected spontaneously.

Disadvantages
- Hospitalization is required for constant monitoring
- Portable X-ray required to look for alignment of bone
- Approximately 20° and there is always slight flexion of both the hip and the knee. The advantage of Russell traction is that some movement in bed is permissible. The patient can turn slightly toward the side in traction for back care, bedpan placement, or linen change.

Precautions while traction in place
- Regular monitoring of pulses
- Check for tape and wrappings
- The foot end of the bed should be elevated to prevent slipping of the patient.

Q14. Write a short note on painful heel.

Ans: Heel pain is one of the most common orthopedic conditions encountered in young adults.

Differential diagnosis includes
- Plantar fasciitis
- Trauma
- Distal tibial tarsal syndrome
- Systemic metabolic disorders like gout, rheumatoid arthritis, etc.
- Calcaneal apophysitis
- Benign and malignant bone tumors
- Fat pad atrophy.

Investigations
- ESR (F), rheumatoid factor, serum uric acid
- *X-rays:* Heel spurs originating from medial calcaneal tuberosity may seen on lateral radiographs of hindfoot.

Treatment
- Treat the cause
- Avoid walking long distances and standing for long periods
- Foot and calf stretching exercises
- NSAIDs
- Cold fomentation
- Use of well fitted shoes
- Orthoptics: Cushioned heel in shoe wear.

Q15. Write a short note on total knee replacement. *(3, DU)*

Ans: Knee replacement is one of the most common performed orthopedic procedures.

Etiology: The most common cause of chronic knee pain and disability is arthritis. Although there are many types of arthritis, most knee pain is caused by just three types:

1. Osteoarthritis.
2. Rheumatoid arthritis.
3. Post-traumatic arthritis.

Indications for knee replacement in cases of arthritis

• Severe knee pain or stiffness that limits your everyday activities.

• Moderate or severe knee pain while resting, either day or night.

• Severe valgus or varus knee deformity.

• Failure to substantially improve with other treatments such as anti-inflammatory medications, cortisone injections, physiotherapy, etc.

Basic steps of knee replacement

a. The damaged cartilage surfaces at the ends of the femur and tibia are removed along with a small amount of underlying bone.

b. The removed cartilage and bone is replaced with metal components that recreate the surface of the joint. These metal parts may be cemented into the bone.

c. A plastic spacer is inserted between two femoral and tibial metal components.

Complications: The complication rate following total knee replacement is low:

• Infection

• Deep vein thrombosis

• Implant may loosen or wear down

• Neurovascular injury.

Chapter 13

Instruments and Implants

1. Osteotome

Identification feature: It has handle with a blade with its surface is bevelled (two sharp surfaces at the end).

Uses

a. For cutting bone (known as osteotomy) like in French osteotomy for malunited supracondylar humerus and McMurray's osteotomy in fracture neck of femur.
b. Creating window in bone (known as saucerization).
c. In bone grafting to harvest the graft from iliac crest.
d. Excising a bony outgrowth (known as exostosis).

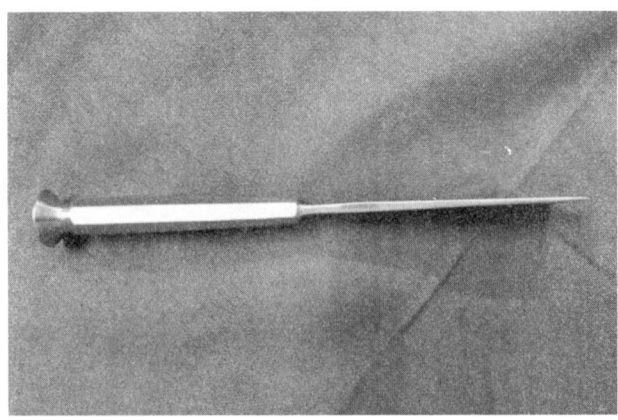

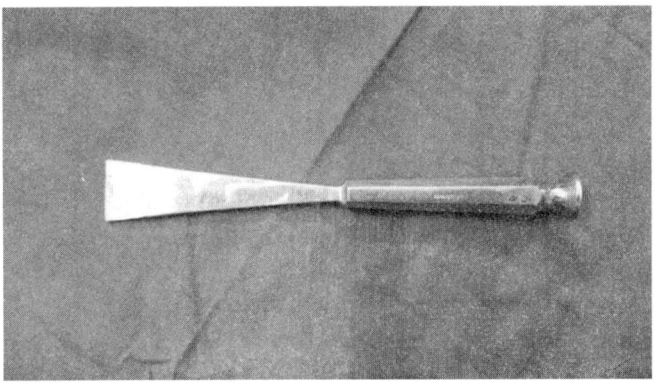

2. Bone Chisel

Identification feature: It has a handle with a blade with only single bevelled (sharp) surface. It is similar in appearance to osteotome except that only one surface is sharp in comparison to both surfaces in osteotome.

Uses

a. Removing a bony outgrowth (osteochondroma or exostosis).

b. Harvesting bone graft from iliac crest.

c. Removing extra callus in hypertrophic non-union.

d. Removing osteophytes.

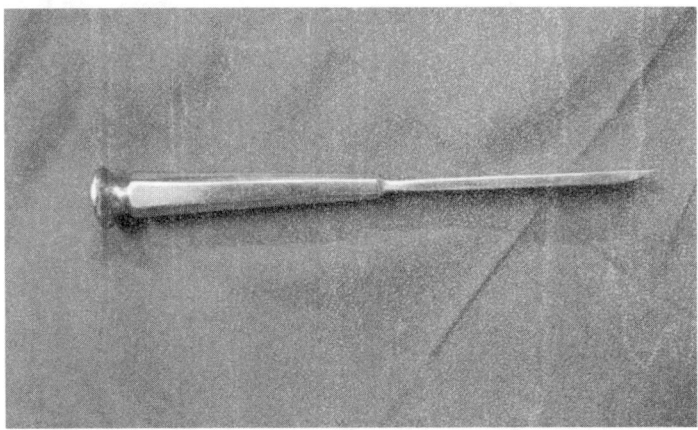

3. Mallet

Identification feature: Stainless hammer with wooden handle (difference from hammer is that later is completely made of stainless steel with no wooden component).

Uses

a. Hammer the bone chisel or osteotome (you can list out all the uses of bone chisel and osteotome).

b. To insert or take out intramedullary nail in tibia or femur.

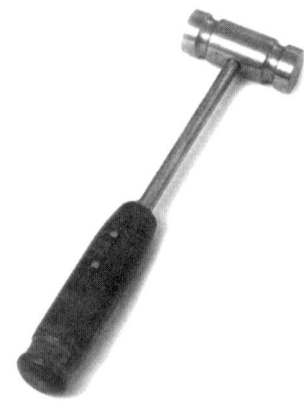

4. Farabeuf's Periosteal Elevator

Identification feature: Stainless steel instrument with flat handle with serrations towards the end to hold with thumb and a straight end with single bevelled surface (like bone chisel).

Use: To strip or lift off periosteum to create a space for application of bone levers thus preventing damage to overlying blood vessels and nerves.

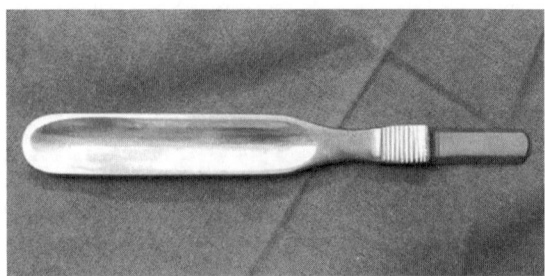

5. Lane's Bone Lever

Identification feature: It has long blunt blade with shank and finger grip. It is smooth and curved at the tip.

Use: It is used to keep the periosteum and other soft tissue away from the operative field (i.e. bone) after elevation of periosteum using periosteal elevator.

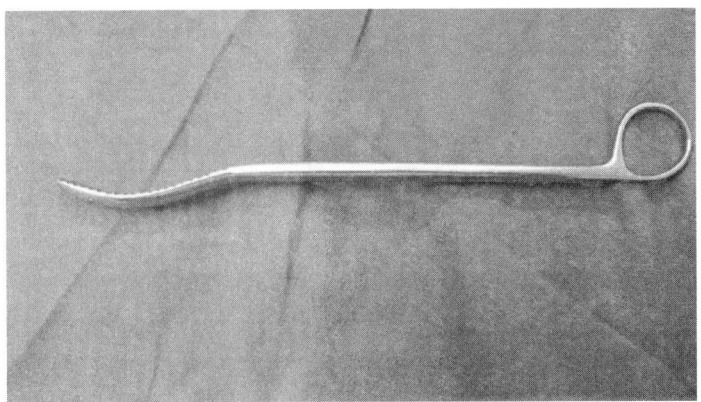

6. Hohmann's Retractor

Identification feature: It has a long hand handle with wide blunt end and a sharp tip.

Use: It allows for retraction of soft tissues away from the operative field especially performing surgeries around the joint.

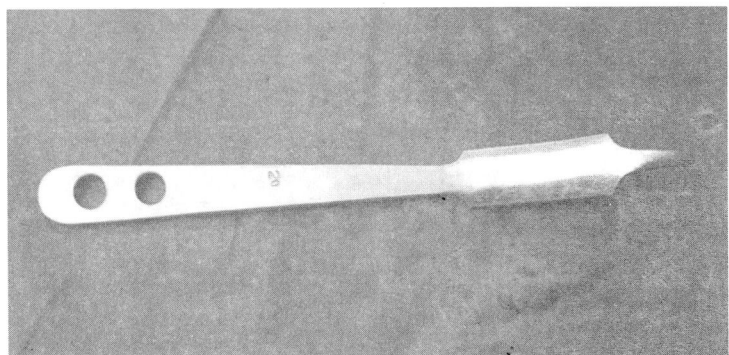

7. Langenbeck Retractor (Right-angled Retractor)

Identification feature: It has a long handle with triangular fenestrations and blunt end bent at right angle.

Use: It allows for retraction of soft tissues away from the operative field.

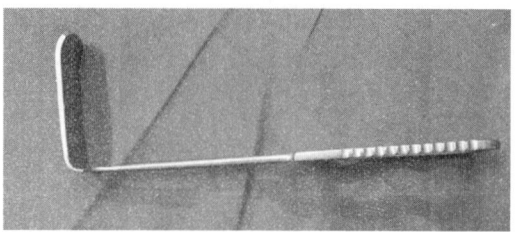

8. Bone Nibbler

Types

 a. Straight nibbler
 b. Curved nibbler
 c. Double action nibbler: It has longer handle with dual hinge which allows bone nibbling with minimal force.

Identification feature: There is nibbler at the end with hinged lever arms separated by tension strip.

Uses

 a. It allows for nibbling for bone as in surgeries involving non-union and malunion.
 b. To remove soft tissue from the bony cavities or from the surface of the bone.
 c. Curved nibbler is used in spine surgeries to remove spinous process of vertebral body.

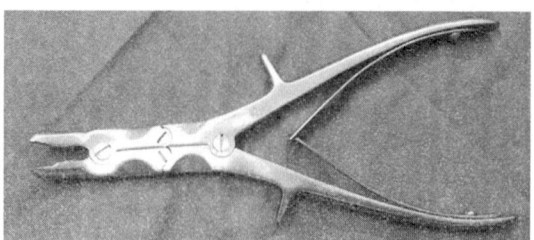

9. Bone Plier

Identification feature: It has stainless steel handle with serrated ends with an eye.

Uses

a. Tighten the wire in tension band wiring for patella and olecranon.

b. Cut Kirschner's wire.

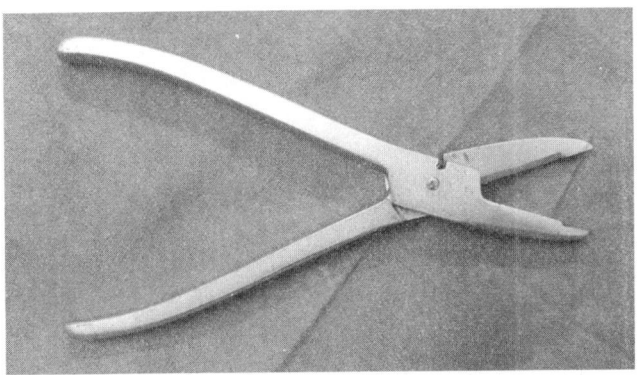

10. Bone Cutter

Identification feature: It has sharp cutting jaws with double-hinged lever arms separated by tension strip.

Use: It is used to cut bone into pieces of desired length and shape. The bone graft harvested from iliac crest is cut into variable sizes and put at the site of non-union of fracture.

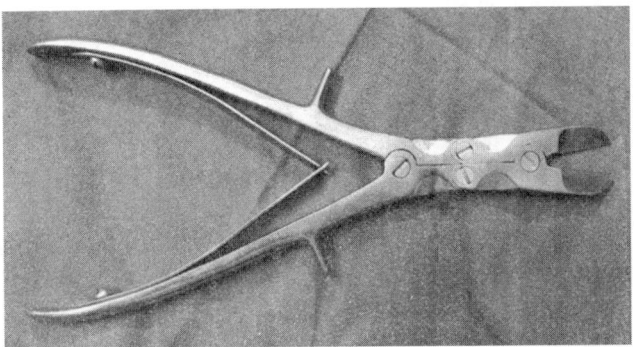

11. Bohler's Stirrup

Identification feature: U-shaped steel rod with two parallel limbs and a twisted base. The ends of parallel limbs are tightened to a Steinman pin and base is attached to the weights with the help of nylon cord.

Use: It is used to apply skeletal traction through proximal tibia, calcaneum and distal femur.

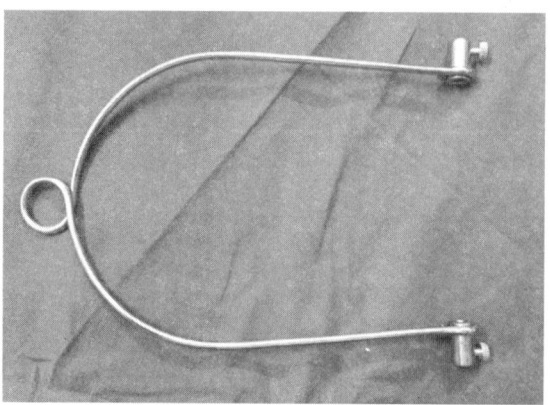

12. Drill Bit

Identification feature: Stainless steel thin rod with spiral twists towards the end with sharp tip.

Uses

   a. Prior to insertion of the screws or pins it is used to create hole in the bone.
   b. Used in osteotomy (it is used to create multiple drill holes in the bone which weakens and helps in cutting the bone).

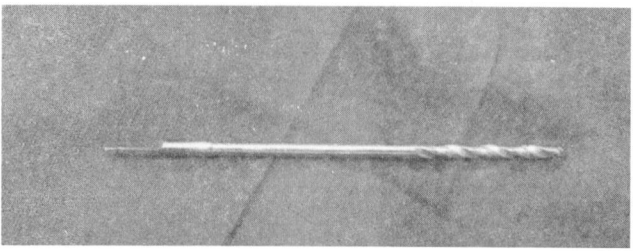

13. Bone Tap

Identification feature: It is a T-shaped stainless steel device with cutting threads at the end.

Use: It is used to create threads in the hole so that the screws can be inserted.

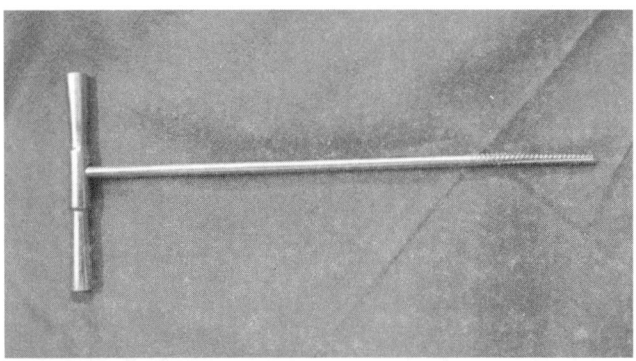

14. Screw Driver

Identification feature: It has a flat wooden handle with steel rod attached to it with hexagonal tip.

Sizes: 3.5 mm and 4.5 mm as per the size of hexagonal tip.

Use: It is used to insert the screws. The screw is mounted/applied over the hexagonal tip and wooden handle is twisted with minimal pressure. The rotatory movements at the wooden handle provide mechanical advantage in terms of less force required to insert a screw in a solid tissue like bone.

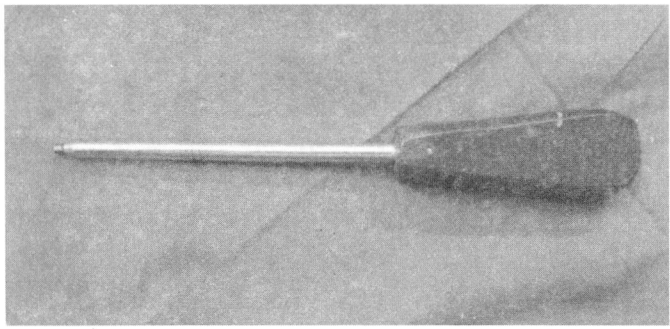

15. Depth Gauge

Identification feature: A sliding rod with bent tip and marking scale on the other end is within the tubular sleeve. The scale moves within the sleeve.

Use: It is used to measure the appropriate size of the screw required to attach the plate with the bone.

Sequence in plate application: Place the palate over bone > drill the hole with drill bit > measure the size of the screw with depth gauge > create threads in the hole > insert the screw of the size measured with depth gauge.

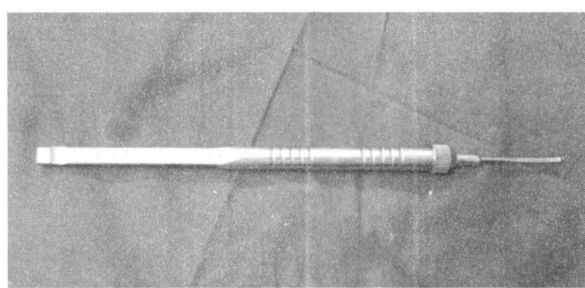

16. Kirschner's Wire

Identification feature: Straight thin stainless steel rods with sharp tip at both the ends.

Size: 1 to 3 mm

Uses

a. For internal fixation of displaced fractures in children like supracondylar humerus, lateral condylar humerus, etc.
b. For internal fixation of fractures of hand and feet in adults.
c. To temporary hold the displaced bony fragments in surgery.

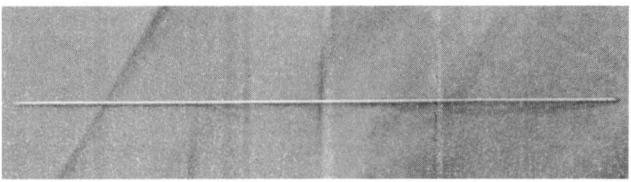

17. Steinmann Pin

Identification feature: Straight stainless rod with sharp tip and triangular end.

Size: 3 to 6 mm.

Uses

1. It is used to apply skeletal traction
2. As a fracture reduction tool in lower limb surgeries.

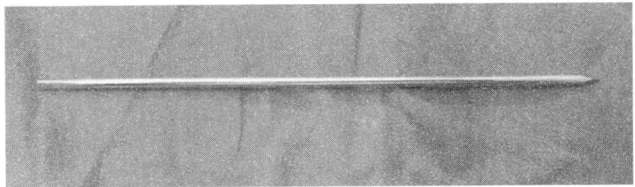

18. Denham's Pin

Identification feature: It is a stainless-steel rod similar in appearance to Steinmann pin with threaded portion in the middle.

Uses

a. To apply skeletal traction through calcaneum
b. As part of external fixator in distal tibia fractures. It is passed through the calcaneum.

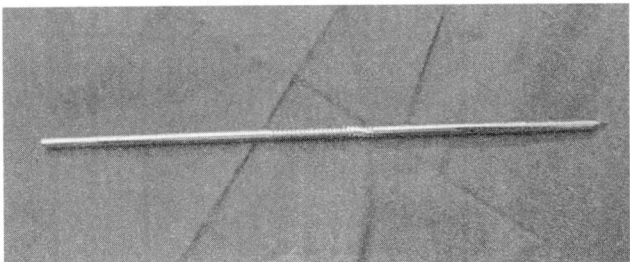

19. Schanz's Pin

Identification feature: It is a stainless-steel rod similar to Steinmann pin with cortical (small threads) or cancellous (larger threads) at the end with sharp tip.

Uses

   a. It is a part external fixator assembly

   b. As a fracture reduction tool.

   c. As a part of Ilizarov's fixator in some selected cases.

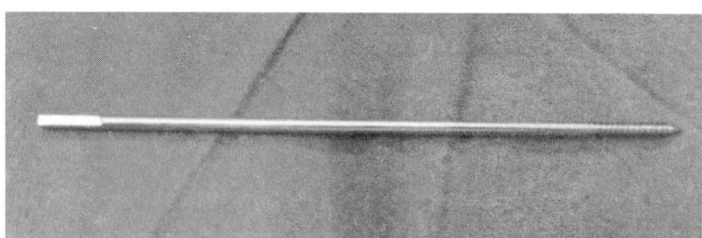

20. Bone Holding or Reduction Forceps

Identification feature: It is stainless forceps serrated with locking mechanism towards the proximal end.

Use: It is used to reduce the fracture by holding its two ends (of course with two bones separate bone holdings).

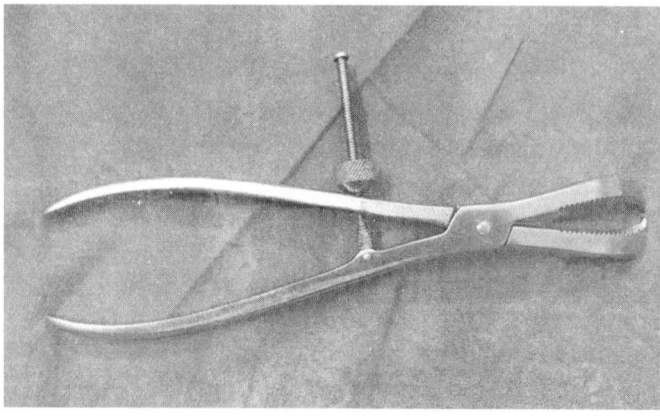

21. Plate Holding Forceps

Identification forceps: It is stainless forceps with bird-like beaked jaw and locking mechanism towards the proximal end.

Use: It is used to hold the plate in place while screws are being applied.

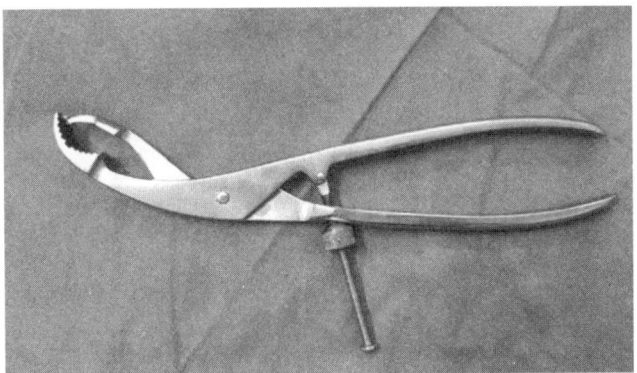

22. Pointed Reduction

Identification feature: It has sharp pointed and curved ends and a proximal lock with the handle.

Use: The intra-articular fractures (fracture extending into joint) around knee and elbow joints are reduced with its help.

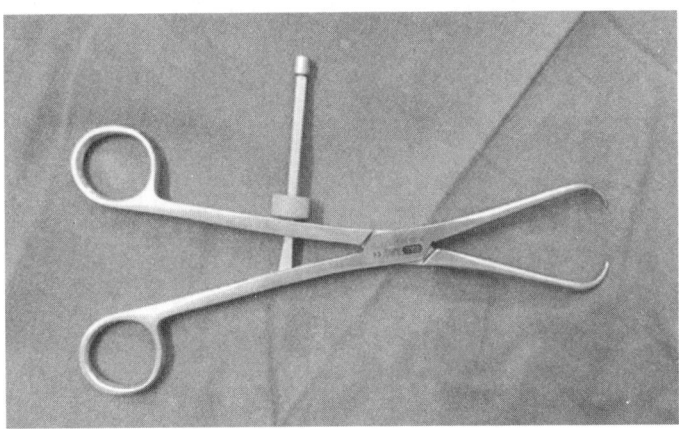

23. Steinmann Pin Holder and Introducer

Identification feature: It has a T-shaped handle at the proximal end with Jacob's chuck at the other end. The Jacob's chuck is tightened with the help of a key.

Use: It is used to hold and introduce Steinmann pin and Schanz pin in bone after drilling the bone.

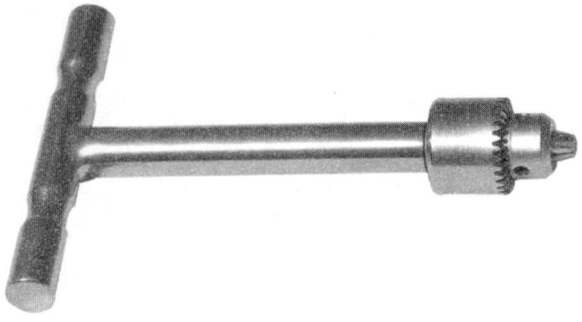

24. Kuntscher's Nail

A famous German surgeon Kuntscher devised the intramedullary nail for fixating femoral shaft fractures.

Identification feature: Straight hollow nail with pointed tip at one end and eye at another end. The extractor is applied over the eye to remove the nail. The nail is cloverleaf in cross section.

Use: It is used in open reduction and internal fixation of femoral and humeral shaft fracture.

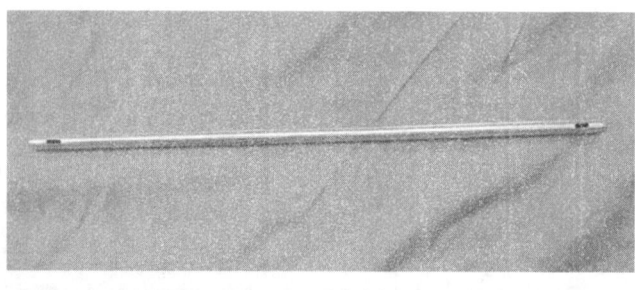

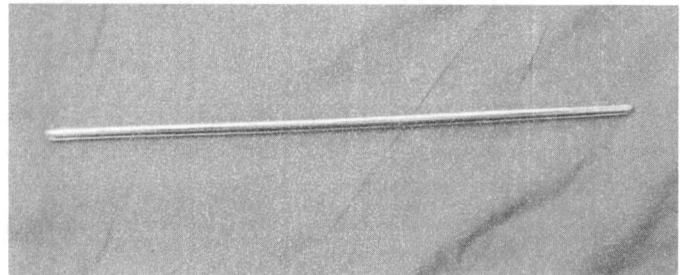

25. Interlocking Nail

Identification feature

a. *Femur interlocking nail:* Straight hollow nail with a mild bow in the middle to match the natural bow of the femur.

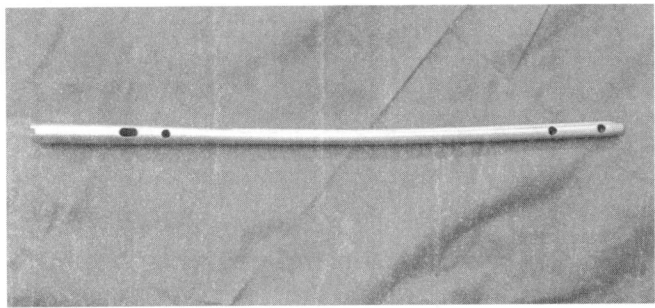

b. *Tibia interlocking nail:* Straight hollow nail with a sharp bend (known as Herzog's bend) at one end.

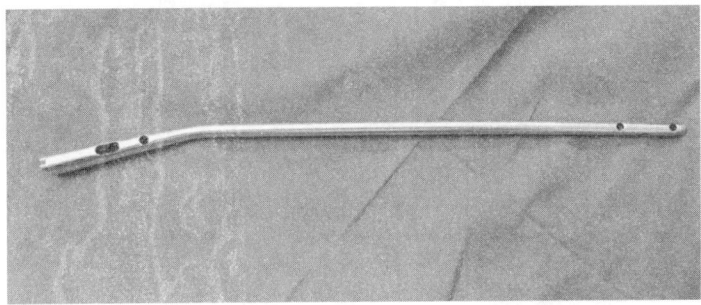

Both nails have two holes at the proximal and distal ends to insert locking bolts. The locking bolts provide rotational stability at the fracture site. Among holes at the ends there are round and elongated holes. The round holes provide the static stability and elongated hole provides the dynamic stability.

Use: Interlocking nails are used for closed or open reduction and internal fixation of shaft fractures of long bones like femur, tibia and humerus. They have the advantage of closed reduction, maintains length of bone, early mobilization and rotational stability over the Kuntscher's nail.

26. Dynamic Hip Screw

Identification feature: It has two components:

a. *Compression hip screw:* It a stainless-steel cannulated rod with threads at one end and rectangular shaft at another end.

b. *Barrel plate:* It has short barrel which is round on outer side and rectangular on inner side to accommodate the compression hip screw. The barrel is attached to plate at an angle of 135°. The plate is applied over the bone with the help of screws.

Both components provide "controlled compression" at the fracture site.

Use: It is used to treat the intertrochanteric fractures, basicervical fracture neck of femur and subtrochanteric fractures.

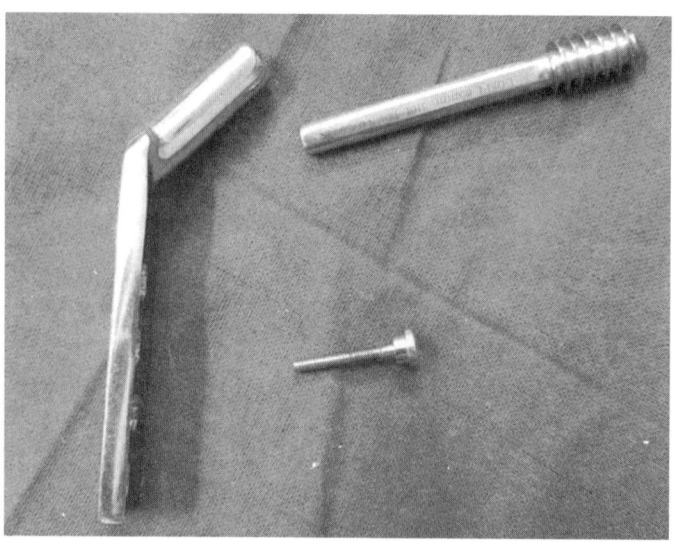

27. Dynamic Compression Plate (DCP)

Identification feature: A flat rigid plate with multiple holes for screws. The holes have a slope in downwards and horizontal direction which helps in compression at the fracture site. The screw slides through these holes when tightened and moves the plate in opposite direction to the fracture site.

Size

a. Broad

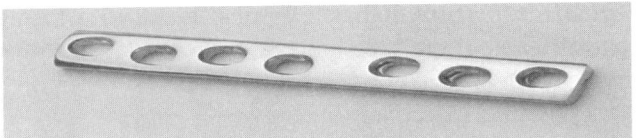

b. Narrow

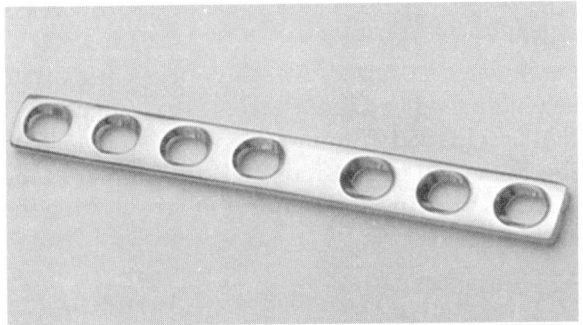

c. Small

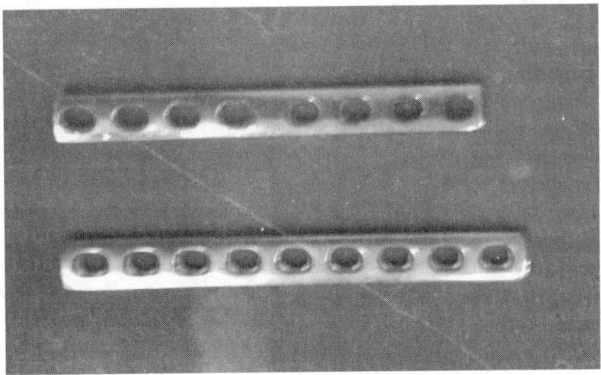

Use: It is used for open reduction and internal fixation of diaphyseal fractures. Broad DCP is used for femur fractures. Narrow DCP is used for humerus and tibia fractures. Small DCP is used for forearm fractures.

28. Screws

Cortical screw

Identification feature: It has spherical head with hexagonal slot and threads along the shaft. The hexagonal slot provides mechanical advantage in terms of lesser pressure required for introduction and extraction of screw.

Uses

a. The plates are applied to bone with the help of cortical screws in the cortical part of bone.

b. It can be used as lag screw when near cortex (part of the bone where the head of the screw is expected to sit) is over drilled or widened in comparison to the other end or cortex of the bone. Due to differential drilling of the bone, the screw tries to bring the two fragments of the bone nearer to each other.

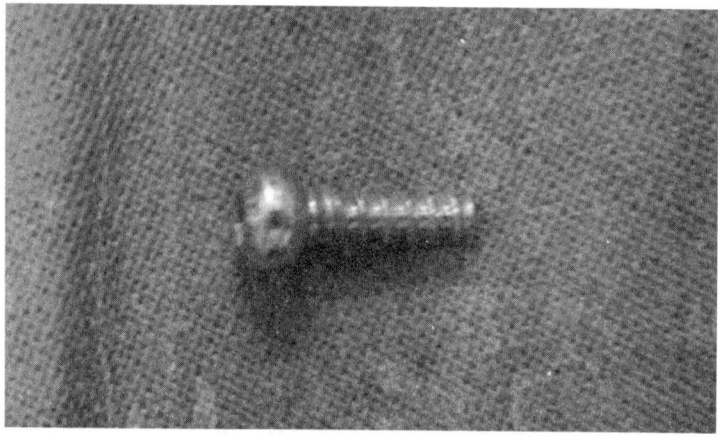

Cancellous Screw

Identification feature: It is like cortical screw except that the pitch or threads are wider spaced and longer in it.

Use: It is used to fix plate to the cancellous or soft part of the bone.

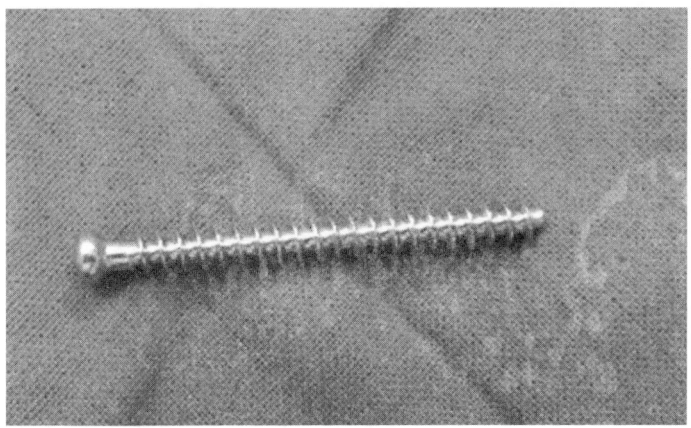

29. Locking Plate

Identification feature: A flat rigid plate with multiple holes for screws. The difference from dynamic compression plate is the presence of threads in the holes of the plate.

Use: It is used in the fixation of osteoporotic fractures and fractures around joint.

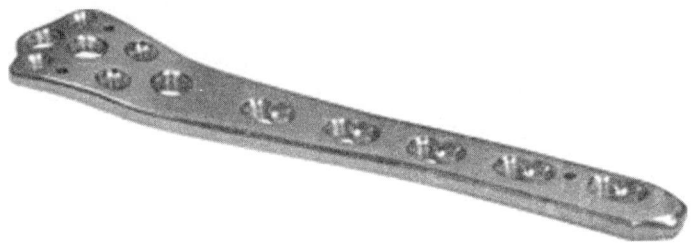

30. Locking Compression Plate

Identification feature: It is a rigid flat plate with two semilunar slots in each hole. One among the two slots has threads which is the locking hole and other has downward and horizontal slope as in dynamic compression plate.

Use: It provides the freedom to surgeon to choose the plate as locking plate or DCP depending upon the fracture type and configuration.

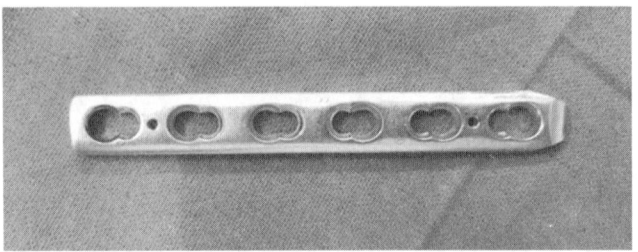

31. Smith Peterson Nail

Identification feature: It is triflanged cannulated nail. Mc Laughlins's plate is applied over the side of proximal femur engaging the nail.

Use: It is used in internal fixation of fracture neck of femur and intertrochanteric fractures.

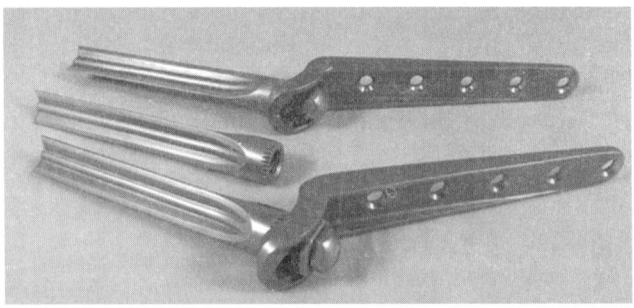

32. Austin Moore Prosthesis

Identification feature: It is stainless steel prosthesis consisting of head, neck and shaft or stem. The head is round with variable sizes ranging from 35 to 55 mm neck has lateral fenestration for extraction or removal of the implant. The stem has two fenestrations in the middle which allows for bone growth and introduction of bone graft. It has a smooth tip which prevents perforation of lateral cortex of femur.

Use: It is used in treatment of fracture of neck of femur in elderly patients where calcar (strong bone over the posteromedial part of the neck connecting with femur shaft) is present. It can be inserted directly or with the help of bone cement in the proximal part of femur in case of osteoporotic bones.

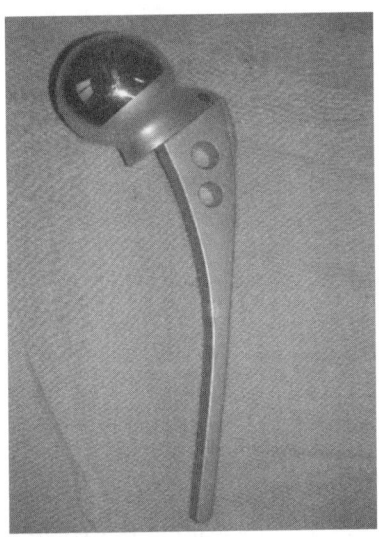

33. Thompson's Prosthesis

Identification feature: It has smooth finish with head, neck and stem or shaft.

Use: It is also used in the treatment of fracture neck of femur in elderly where calcar is less than 2.5 cm. It is fixed exclusively with the help of bone cement.

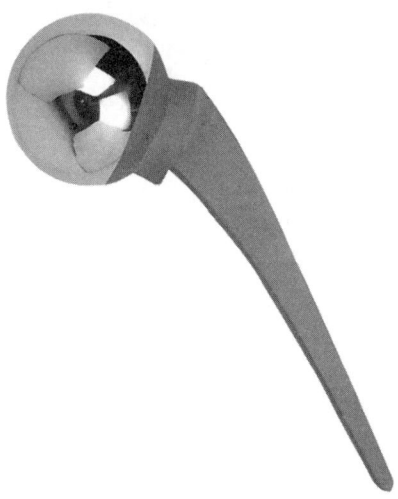

34. Charnley's Total Hip Prosthesis

It was developed by Sir John Charnley—the father of total hip replacement.

Identification feature: It has three components—metallic head, stem and polyethylene cup. The metallic head and stem is made of steel. The diameter of head is 22 mm. The head and stem is fixed to the femur and polyethylene cup is fixed to acetabulum with bone cement (polymethyl-methacrylate).

Uses

1. Avascular necrosis of femoral head leading to osteoarthritis of hip joint.
2. Selected cases of neglected neck of femur.
3. Primary osteoarthritis of hip joint.
4. Neglected cases of developmental dysplasia of hip presenting in adulthood.

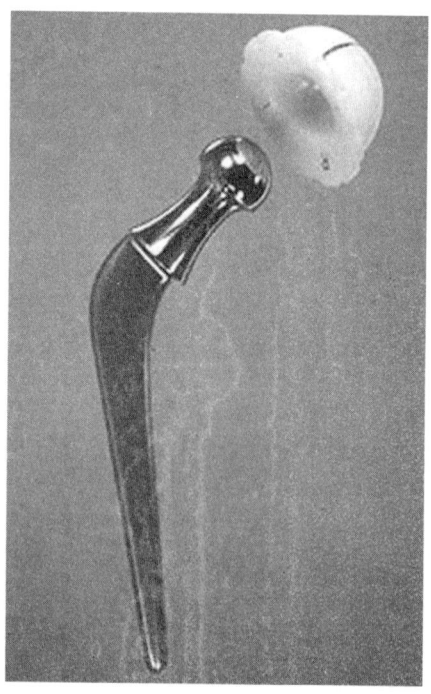

35. Crutch Field or Skull Traction Tongs

Identification feature: It has two stainless steel tongs with pointed tips and a proximal locking mechanism.

Use: It is used to apply traction to the cervical spine by pulling through skull in cases of cervical spine injury or diseases and in some cases of cervical spine injury before performing surgery.

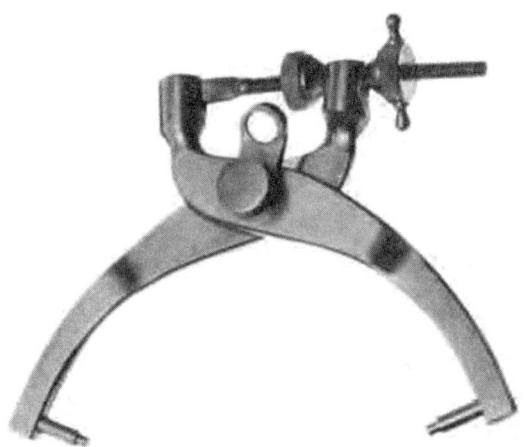

36. Bone Gouge

Identification feature: It has stainless steel handle with a semitubular blade and a sharp edge.

Uses

    a. To clear bony cavities of tissue.

    b. Harvest bone graft.

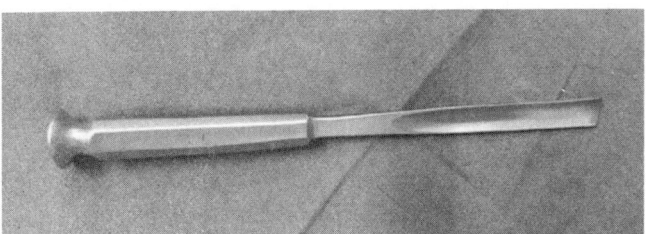

37. Bone Awl

Identification feature: It has U-shaped handle with curved shaft and a pointed tip.

Use: It is used to make entry point through which the nails can be introduced into the medullary canals of the long bones.

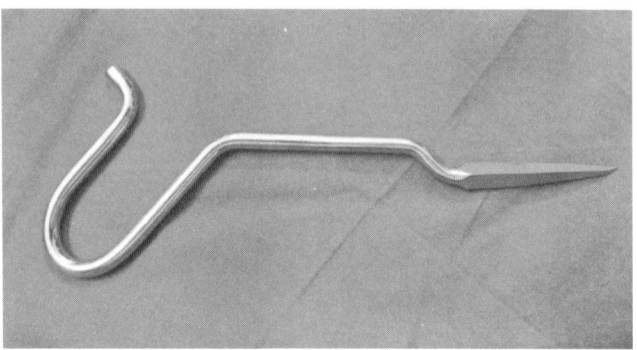

38. Bone Curette

Identification feature: It has flat handle with serrations and small cups at two ends. The cups are of different sizes.

Uses

a. It is used to curette out tissue from bony cavities which may be due to tumor, bone infection.

b. To freshen the fracture margins.

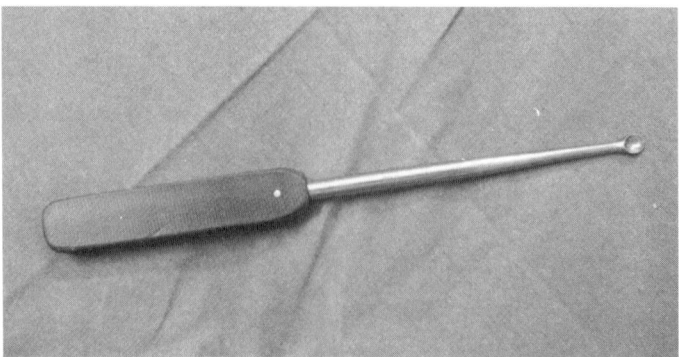

39. External Fixator

It has the following components:

a. *Tubular rod:* It is stainless steel horizontal tubular rod varying in length from 10 to 45 cm.

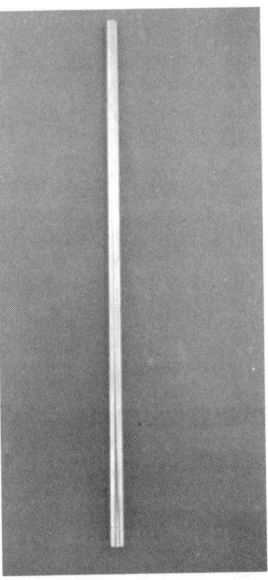

b. *Universal clamp:* It has two slots, smaller one holds the Shanz pin and tubular rod passes through the bigger one. It connects Shanz pin to the tubular rod.

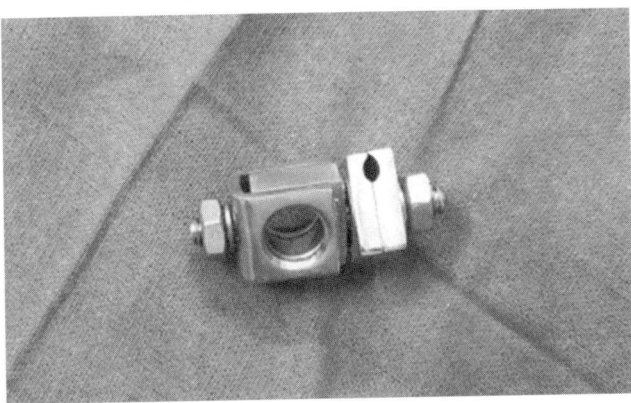

c. Schanz pin

Uses

1. It is used in the primary management of compound fractures.
2. It is used in the preliminary management of complex closed periarticular fractures.
3. In managing extensive soft tissue injuries.
4. As a supportive fixation device in extensively comminuted fractures.

40. Ilizarov's Ring Fixator

It was designed by professor GA Ilizarov. He was famously known as "magician of Kurgan"—a place in Russia.

Components

1. *Ring:* Stainless steel rings measuring between 80 and 240 mm with holes in it. The two rings are connected by small bolts converting into a full ring.

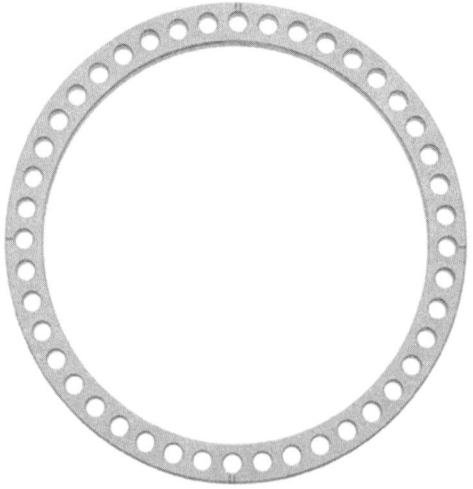

2. *K-wire:* They are specially designed with diameter 1.5 to 1.8 mm.
3. *Threaded rods:* Stainless steel threaded rods with a diameter of 6 mm.

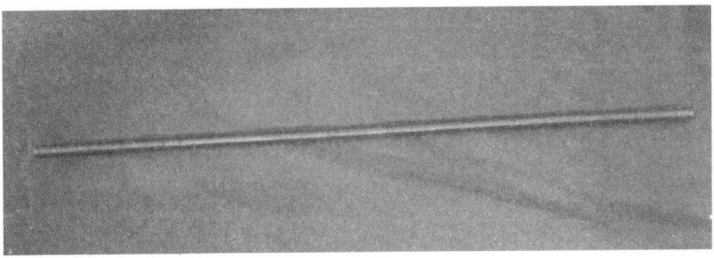

Uses

  a. Limb lengthening on principle of distraction histogenesis.

  b. Treatment of displaced comminuted fractures.

  c. Arthrodesis

  d. Deformity correction.

Index